AN OVERVIEW OF REPERTORIES
for PG Students

Dr. D.P. Rastogi
D.M.S., M.B.S., DF Hom., M.D. Hom.

Director
Boenninghausen Academy for Classical Homeopathy
Director PG Studies,
SKH Medical College, Beed.

Second Edition

B. Jain Publishers (P) Ltd.
An ISO 9001 : 2000 Certified Company
USA – Europe – India

AN OVERVIEW OF REPERTORIES
for PG Students

First Edition : 2004
Second Edition : 2008

© Copyright with the Publishers

All rights are reserved. No part of this book may be reproduced, stored in a retrieval system or transmitted, in any form or by any means, mechanical, photocopying, recording or otherwise, without any prior written permission of the publishers.

Published by Kuldeep Jain for
B. Jain Publishers (P) Ltd.
1921, Street No. 10, Chuna Mandi, Paharganj,
New Delhi–110 055 (INDIA)
Ph.: 91-11-2358 0800, 2358 3100, 2358 1300, 2358 1100
Fax: 91-11-2358 0471 • **Email:** bjain@vsnl.com
Website: www.bjainbooks.com

Printed in India by
J.J. Offset Printers
522, FIE, Patpar Ganj, Delhi–110092
Ph.: 91-11-2216 9633, 2215 6128

ISBN : 978-81-319-0329-2

Preface to First Edition

Several of my students have urged me to write a book on repertory. Honestly, in the first go I did not feel the need to undertake this work, as there are several books already available on the subject. However, on persistent demands, I agreed to publish an article that has proved informative and useful to students. It was published in the souvenir of the HMAI's conference in Bangalore in the year 1998. In response to the article I received many queries and I realised that book should come out for all the queries thus the project started. I have taken care to update it with more data so that at one glance it may give on overview of repertory development and open the door for detailed study.

In my experience as a teacher, guide and examiner of repertory, I have come across repeated spelling mistakes in the books available on the subject as well as mistakes committed by students. I would ask the students to check on this. Often I have found the following mis-spelled:

Jahr as Jhar

Clarke as Clark

Hering as Herring or Hearing

Roger Van Zandvoort is hardly correctly spelt

Boenninghausen being spelt as Bonning Hussain

Knerr as Kneer

Boger as Bogar

Lamnia as Lamina

Phatak as Pathak

Dr. Gross as Dr. Grass

In the various books available to the students, there are numerous errors in the year of publication and number of drugs included in a particular repertory besides aforesaid spelling mistakes. An example can be given of the year of publication of the first edition of Kent's Repertory, instead of the correct year of publication as 1897 it is mentioned as 1857. I would like to caution the students to be careful on this and double check the data. Needless to say that our authors have a greater responsibility towards including verified data and avoiding awful spelling mistakes of the names of the creators of repertory in the next editions of their works.

I hope this small write up would be informative and generate interest in repertories.

I would like to thank Dr. Subhash Arora and Dr. Anil Singhal for their assistance. Thanks are also due to Kusum for computer setting.

Dr. D.P. Rastogi

Preface to Second Edition

This is indeed gratifying to note that this small book has served the purpose for which it was written. It has been of great help to students preparing for examination. I have tried to incorporate more information about repertories in this edition besides updating the write-ups of the earlier edition with current information. I hope it will prove of immense benefit to students.

I would like to thank both my students Dr. Suresh Barik and Dr. Arindam Dutta for assisting me in adding material in clinical repertories, Bonninghausen's concordances and selected clinical rubrics in BBCR. I would also like to thank Dr. Harpreet Kaur for carefully checking the manuscript. I am sure these additions would interest the readers to use BTPB and BBCR more profitably.

Dr. D.P. Rastogi
March 2007

Introduction

The totality of symptoms in contrast to pathology plays the key role in understanding a drug or patient in homeopathy. The selection of the simillimum from vast symptomatology of materia medica always demands some way of differentiating or sorting out similar looking drugs, and repertorization is one such comprehensive, scientific and precise tool of accomplishing this.

The root of repertory idea can be traced to as early as 1816 to the preamble of *Materia Medica Pura* by Hahnemann himself who wrote, "For the convenience of treatment, we require merely to jot down after each symptom all the medicines which can produce such a symptom with tolerable accuracy, expressing them by a few letters (abbreviations) and also to bear in mind the circumstances under which they occur, they have a determining influence on our choice, and proceed in the same way with all the other symptoms, noting by which medicine each is excited from the list so prepared we shall be able to perceive which among the medicines homeopathically covers most of the symptoms present, especially the most peculiar and characteristic ones and this is the remedy sought for." This laid the foundation of the present day repertories.

From the first repertory *Fragmenta De Viribus Medica Mentorum Positivis Sive in Sano Corpore Humano Observatis* published in 1805 by Hahnemann himself, the profession has seen a large number of repertories and the search for an ideal and complete repertory will go on unabated in future.

The credit for publishing the first repertory goes to von Boenninghausen. Boenninghausen published Repertory of the Antipsorics in 1832 with a preface by the master (second edition in 1833). *Hahnemann himself in his practice used this repertory.* In the preface to the second edition, Boenninghausen says about undertaking a rigorous revision of the first edition. This shows his remarkable accuracy.

In 1835, *Boenninghausen's Repertory of Medicines Which are Not–Antipsorics* and in 1836 *An Attempt at Showing the Relative Kinship of Homeopathic Medicines* was published. All these publications were combined to form his masterpiece the Therapeutic Pocket Book (TPB) which was published in 1846 in German. This became the standard reference work used by most American Homeopaths including Stuart Close, Carroll Dunham, H.N. Guernsey and T.F. Allen. Even Dr. Kent used this for 20 years.

Recently this book has come in to great use and new editions have appeared in German and English by Dr. Gypser and Dimitriadis that are based on the original *'Therapeutisches Taschenbuch'*, (TT). These editions are praiseworthy as they are based on the original book rather than on the translations made by people like A.H. Okie, C.J. Hempel and J. Laurie. Besides it has taken care to correct T.F. Allen's error in respect of the 5 gradations (ranks) of remedies instead of Bonninghausen's 4. The number of remedies added to the original copy of Boenninghausen by Dr. T.F. Allen have been deleted leaving behind only 125 remedies as these were not found consistent with Boenninghausen's plan. The English edition has been done by G. Dimitriadis, Sydney in the year 2000 and is known as *The Boenninghausen Repertory* (TBR).

In 1900, Cyrus Maxwell Boger made a new translation of the Antipsoric Remedies into English. It contained 232 pages. This repertory later grew into Boger Boenninghausen's Characteristics and Repertory and was published in 1905. He made so many additions and added new rubrics that its final size was 1040 pages an almost five fold increase. Dr. Boger continued to enhance it until his death in 1935.

Contents

Historical Development of Repertories 1
    Regional and Clinical Repertories 5
    Card Repertories 8
    Number of Remedies in each Repertory 9
    Types of Repertory based on the Philosophy
    of Construction 10

Details of Some Lesser Known and Latest Repertories 25
    Boenninghausen's Repertories 25
    Boger Boenninghausen's Repertory – 1905 35
    Knerr's Repertory – 1896 68
    Thematic Repertory by J.A. Mirrili – 1995 70
    Robin Murphy's Repertory of Homeopathic
        Materia Medica Released in March 1993 71
    Complete Repertory by Roger Van Zandvoort 77
    Synthesis: Repertorium Homeopathicum
        Syntheticum by Frederik Schroyens 80
    Gentry's Repertory 82
    Integrated Homoeopathic Repertory of Mind by
        Dr. J. Kishore 85
    Integrated Homoepathic Repertory of Generalities
        by Dr. Jugal Kishore 86
    Mini Repertories 87

Some Clinical Repertories 88

Computerized Repertories 93
    RADAR (Rapid Aid to Drug Aimed Research) of Windows
    Version 6 and Encyclopedia Homeopathica (EH) 93
    Reference works 99
    CARA & SIMILIA 100
    Hompath 101
    Homeopathic Repertorization System (HRS) 104
    Phoenix Repertory 105
    Phatak's Repertory 106
    Kentian Homeopathic Computer Programme 106
    ISISV2 107

Corrections of Abbreviations for Medicines
Used in Boger-Boenninghausen's Repertory 109

Appendix
    Books in Encyclopedia Homeopathica Software 134
    Books in Reference Works Library 174
    CARA Professional 198

HISTORICAL DEVELOPMENT OF REPERTORIES

1805 **Fragmenta de Viribus Medica Mentorum Positivis Sive in Sano Corpore Humano Observatis** by Hahnemann.

1828 Hartlaub's **Repertory** in Leipzig.

1830 Systematiche Dartellung der Antipsorische Arzneimittal By Weber In German consisting of 536 pages.

1832 Boenninghausen's **Repertory of the Antipsorics** with a preface by Hahnemann.

1833 Weber-Peschier's **Repertory of Purely Pathogenetic Effects** prefaced by Hahnemann consisting of 376 pages.

1835 **Jahr's Repertory** – work assigned by Dr. Hahnemann. It was published in two volumes consisting of 1052 and 1254 pages in German.

Another repertory of 200 pages – on glands, bones, mucous membrane, ducts and skin diseases.

1835 Boenninghausen's **Repertory of Medicines Which Are Not Antipsoric**

1836 Boenninghausen's **An Attempt at Showing the Relative Kinship of Homeopathic Medicines.**

1837 Ruoff's **Repertory** published in Stuttgart consisting of 236 pages.

1838 **A Repertory** published in English language in Allentown Academy by C. Hering. It was based on the translation of Jahr's Manual.

1840	Ruoff's **"A Repertory of Nosology"** consisting of 250 pages, translated from German by Okie, Humphry and published in English in America.
1843	**A Homoeopathic Repertory of Symptomatology** (first original repertory in French) consisting of 975 pages was published by Laffitte – one of the first Parisian homeopaths.
1846	Boenninghausen's famous **Therapeutic Pocket Book.** It was translated in English by Dr. Hempel, Dr. J. Laurie and also by Dr. Okie. Later Dr. T.F. Allen published another edition with modification. The last and current edition was published by Dr. H.A. Roberts of Connecticut, U.S.A. in 1935, who also edited and made some modifications in it.
1847	**Hempel's Boenninghausen Repertory** consisting of 500 pages.
1847	Jahr's **Manual of Homoeopathic Materia Medica and Repertory** edited by P.F. Curie.
1848	Clotar Muller's **Systematic Alphabetical Repertory** consisting of 940 pages.
1849	Mure's [Rio de Janeiro] consisting of 367 pages.
1851	Bryant's (New York) an alphabetical repertory **"A Pocket Manual of Repertory of Homeopathic Medicine"** consisting of 367 pages. It was made especially for laymen.
1853	Possart's **A Repertory of Characteristic Homoeopathic Remedies** consisting of 700 pages, published at Kothen.
1853	**Dysentery and Its Repertory of Medicine** by Fred Humphreys.
1854	Adolph Lippe's (USA) **A Repertory of Comparative Materia Medica** consisting of 144 pages.
1859	**Cipher Repertory** consisting of 600 pages by English homeopaths. Enlarged edition in 1878 containing 1030 pages by Drysdale, Atkins, Dudgeon and Stokes.

1859	Jahr's **New Manual of Homoeopathic Materia Medica with Possart's Additions** – fifth edition revised and enlarged by the author and translated and edited by Hempel.

About this time in England the following repertories were known:
- Buck's **Regional Symptomatology and Clinical Dictionary.**
- **Hempel's Repertory.**
- Curie's **Repertory** by Drysdale and Dudgeon.

1873	Berridge **"Repertory of the Eyes"**, published in England.
1874	Granier of Nimes **Homoeolexicon** in two volumes
1876	**Repertory of the New Remedies** by C.P. Hart published by Boericke and Tafel. Based on Hale's Special Symptomatology and Therapeutics.
1879	C. Lippe published his famous **Repertory of the More Characteristic Symptoms of the Materia Medica** consisting of 322 pages (Indian edition has 438 pages). It became one of the precursors of Kent's Repertory which was published in 1897.
1880	T.F. Allen's **Symptom Register.**
1880	**Repertory to the Modalities** by Samuel Worcester.
1881	Hering's **Analytical Repertory** (Symptoms of the Mind).
1883	**Repertory of Intermittent Fever** by William A. Allen.
1884	**Cough and Expectoration** by Lee and Clarke (first edition). Second edition was published in 1894.
1885	**Alphabetical Repertory** by Father Muller (first repertory published in India).
1888	**Pathogenetic and Clinical Repertory of the Symptoms of Head** by Neidhard.

1890	Gentry's **The Repertory of Concordances** in six volumes – 5500 pages.
1890	**Classified Index of the Materia Medica for Urogenital and Venereal Diseases** by Carleton and Coles.
1896	Knerr's **Repertory to the Hering's Guiding Symptoms.**
1897	Kent's **Repertory of the Homoeopathic Materia Medica** (first edition) consisted of 1349 pages.
1900	Boger's English translation of **Boenninghausen's Repertory of Antipsoric Remedies.**
1905	**Boger Boenninghausen's Characteristics and Repertory.**
1908	**Clinical Repertory** by P.W. Shedd.
1920	Repertory section of **Bell's Diarrhoea.**
1931	**Synoptic Key of the Homoeopathic Materia Medica** by C.M. Boger.
1935-1937	Second and enlarged edition of the **Characteristics and Repertory** by C.M. Boger – **Boger's Times of remedies and Moon Phases** published by Roy & Co. of Bombay.
1929	N.M. Chaudhary's **Materia Medica and Repertory.**
	Piere's **Materia Medica and Repertory.**
1963	**Phatak's Repertory,** 2nd edition in 1977.
1963	**A Materia Medica and Repertory** by James Stephenson.
1973	**Synthetic Repertory** edited by H. Barthel in 3 volumes covering: • Mental Symptoms • Generalities • Sleep, Dreams and Sexuality .
1974	Additions to Kent's repertory by George Vithoulkas.
1980	The **Final General Repertory of Kent** by Diwan Harishchand and Pierre Schmidt.
1983	**Repertory of Psychic Medicines with Materia Medica**

by Dr. Emm Gallavardin translated into English from original French by Dr. Rajkumar Mukerji.

1984   Sharma's **Card Repertory.**

1987   **Kent's General Repertory** by Kunzli. It is regarded as very reliable.

1987   **Synthesis – Repertorium Homoeopathicum Syntheticum** by Dr. Frederik Schroyens.

1990   **Kent's General Repertory** by Kunzli.

1993   **A Modern alphabetical Repertory** by Robin Murphy.

1993   **Clinical Repertories of New Homoeopathic Remedies** by O.A. Julian.

1996   **Complete Repertory** by Roger Van Zandvoort.

1999   **Millennium Repertory** by Roger Van Zandvoort.

1999   **Phoenix Repertory** by J.P.S. Bakshi.

2000   **Integrated Repertory** (Mind chapter) by Jugal Kishore.

2003   **Repertorium Universalis** by Roger Van Zandvoort.

2006   **Integrated Homeopathic Repertory on Generalities** by Jugal Kishore.

REGIONAL AND CLINICAL REPERTORIES

Apart from the above repertories, there were a host of regional and clinical repertories published in America and elsewhere:

1873   **Repertory of Eyes** by Berridge.

          Desires and Aversions by Guernsey.

1879   **Illustrated Repertory (of Pain in chest, sides and back)** by Rolin R. Gregg.

1880   **Repertory of Modalities** by Worcester.

          Repertory of Hemorrhoids by Guernsey.

          Repertory of Respiratory Organs by Lutze.

          Repertory of Fevers by H.C. Allen.

          Repertory of Foot Sweat by O.M. Drake.

1883	**Repertory of Intermittent Fevers** by W.A. Allen.
1884	**Repertory of Cough and Expectoration** by Lee and Clarke.
1888	**Repertory of the Head** by Niedhard.
1890	**Classified Index of Homoeopathic Materia Medica for Urogenital and Venereal Diseases** by Carleton and Coles.
1891	**Headache – Concise Repertory** by King.
1892	**Repertory of Digestive System** by Arkell Mc. Michell.
1894	**Repertory of Rheumatism** by Perkins.
	Repertory of Therapeutics of Respiratory System by Van Denbug.
	Repertory of Eczema by C.F. Mills Paugh.
	Repertory of Headache by Knerr.
	Repertory of the Appendicitis by Yingling.
	Repertory of Headaches by Neatby Stonham.
	Repertory of the Labour by Yingling.
1895	**Repertory of Spasms and Convulsions** by Holcomb.
1896	**Repertory of the Tongue** by Douglass.
1896	**Repertory of the Neuralgia** by Lutze.
1896	**Therapeutics of the Eye** by Charles C. Boyle.
1899	**Repertory of Urinary Organs and Prostate Gland** by A.R. Morgan.
1900	**Repertory of the Back** by Wilsey.
1904	**A Clinical Repertory to the Dictionary of Materia Medica** by John Henry Clarke.
1906	**Repertory of the Uterine Therapeutics** by Minton.
	Repertory by P.F. Curie.
	Repertory Part of Rau's Special Pathology.

Repertory by O.E. Boericke.
Repertory by Dr. Sarkar.
Repertory of Respiratory Diseases by E.B. Nash.
Clarke's **Clinical Repertory.**
Repertory of Mastitis by W.J. Guernsey.
Repertory of Throat by W.J. Guernsey.

1908 **Shedd's Clinical Repertory.**
1920 **Repertory of Diarrhoea** by Bell.
1931 **Boger's Repertory of Times of Remedies and Moon Phases.**
1937 **Repertory of Sensation As If** by Dr. H.A. Roberts.
1945 **Repertory of Rheumatic Remedies** by Dr. H. A. Roberts.

J.W. Ward's Dictionary of Sensation As If (Two volumes).
Repertory of the Digestive Symptom by Michell.
Repertory Section of Homoeopathic Therapeutics of Uterine and Vaginal Discharges by W. Eggert.
Leucorrhea and its Concomitant Symptoms by A.M. Cushing.
Repertory of the Warts in Skin Diseases by Drake.
Repertory of Homoeopathic Therapeutics in Ophthalmology by J. L. Moffat.
Repertory of Convulsions by E. M. Santee.
A Repertory of the Peculiar Symptoms Based on Periodic Drug Disorders by L. Slazer revised by N. K. Banerjee.

CARD REPERTORIES

1. **Dr. William Jefferson Guernsey** nephew of H. N. Guernsey made a repertory in 1888. It was based on Boenninghausen's work. (Also made repertory on Hemorrhoids, Urticaria, Throat, Diphtheria and Mastitis.) It was known as:
   - "**Guernsey's Boenninghausen's Slips**"
   - Long cards of 13.5" in length and 1.5" width.
   - 2500 cards.
   - Contained only 126 remedies.

2. **Dr. H. C. Allen** improved upon the above slips. These were known as **Allen's Boenninghausen Slips**.

3. 1912 – **Dr. Margaret Tyler** created a **Punched Card Repertory** based on Kent's Repertory. It was not approved by Dr. Kent as, in his opinion it would lead to keynote prescribing.

4. 1913 – **Welch and Houston** made a **Loose – Punched Card Repertory** based on Kent's. It contained 134 symptoms.

5. 1922 – **Dr. Field** made a **Gigantic Card Repertory**, having 6800 cards. It was mainly based on Kent's repertory. It contained 360 remedies with a provision for 40 more.

6. 1928 – **Dr. Boger** made a **Card Repertory** which was published by Roy & Co. of Bombay with a foreword from late Dr. L. D. Dhawale.

7. 1948 – George Broussalion's Card Repertory with 640 remedies and 1861 cards.

8. 1948 – Dr. Marcoz Jamenez with 480 remedies and 552 cards.

9. 1950 – **Dr. J.G. Weiss & Dr. Robert H. Farley's**

Spindle's Card Repertory with 274 remedies and 190 cards.

10. 1955 – **Dr. P. Sankaran's Card Repertory** with 420 cards and 292 remedies.

11. **Kishore's Card Repertory**
    - 3500 cards – first edition in 1959.
    - 10,000 cards – second edition in 1967 including six hundred remedies.
    - Third edition in 1986 with more rubrics and remedies.
    - This is the best card repertory available to the profession as it contains a large number of rubrics from Boenninghausen also.

NUMBER OF REMEDIES IN EACH REPERTORY

S. No.	Repertory	Remedies
1.	Boenninghausen's Repertory (TPB)	342
2.	Kent's Repertory	642
3.	Boger Boenninghausen's Characteristics and Repertory	464
4.	Synthetic Repertory	1594
5.	Kishore's Card Repertory	693
6.	Boericke's Repertory	1407
7.	Synthesis Repertory, version 9.1	2373
8.	Knerr's Repertory	408
9.	Complete Repertory	2171
10.	Phoenix Repertory	1607
11.	J.H. Clarke's Repertory	1067
12.	Bell's Diarrhea	141
13.	Symptom Register by Timothy Field Allen	820
14.	The Concordance Repertory of the More Characteristic Symptoms of the Materia Medica by William D. Gentry	420
15.	Homeopathic Medical Repertory by Murphy	1602

TYPES OF REPERTORY BASED ON THE PHILOSOPHY OF CONSTRUCTION

1. Based on the Philosophic Concept of Totality of Symptoms

Boenninghausen's Repertories:

It included:
- Repertory of Antipsorics – 1832.
- Therapeutic Pocket Book – 1846.
- Boger's Boenninghausen's Characteristics and Repertory– 1905.
- Repertory with Synoptic Key by Boger – 1931.

2. Concept of General, Peculiar and Particular Symptoms

  i. **Constantine Lippe's Repertory of More Characteristic Symptoms of the Materia Medica:**

  Constantine Lippe was the son of Adolf Lippe. This repertory was published in the year 1879. It is based on Hering's repertory published in 1838 by Allentown Academy. Hering's repertory was a translation of Jahr's Manual. It also included some additions from Hering, H.N. Guernsey, Adolph Lippe and Boenninghausen.

  This repertory is one of the precursors to Kent's Repertory and contains 301 remedies.

  ii. **Lee's Repertory:**

  This repertory was published in 1889. Dr. Edmund Jennings Lee's Repertory of Mind and Head are based on unreleased second edition of C. Lippe's repertory and from notes and additions from other homoeopaths including E.W. Berridge of England and J.T. Kent of United States. However Lee became blind and his unfinished manuscripts were given to Kent who continued to work on them.

iii. **Kent's repertory—its construction, arrangement of rubrics and utility.**

Kent's Repertory is one of the most known and often used repertory, so much so that the word repertory has almost become synonymous with Kent's repertory. It is regarded as a Gold standard. All modern repertories have taken Kent as the base for additions of more rubrics and drugs. However many do not know how to use it and hence are not able to take advantage of this most useful repertory.

Let us briefly get acquainted with its contents

Finding the rubric in Kent's repertory is often tricky.

For example: If you need to find a rubric *"chilly"* patient you have to look for *"heat vital lack of"* and so on. Speech rubrics are given both under 'Mouth' and 'Mind' chapters.

Once I had a case who never spoke the truth, I tried to look up this under Mind chapter under "t" but it was not to be found there. It is given under *"Lies, never speaks the truth"*.

We have to remember that Kent had a difficult task of creating a repertorial language. To be able to repertorize on Kent's repertory we have to evaluate the symptoms as per Kent's scheme. Selecting rubrics just consisting of common symptoms would not give us the desired result and will often lead to failure in looking up the curative remedy.

Rubrics to be taken in the following order **for use of Kent's repertory.**

- **Characteristics**
    —Will (with loves, hates, fears)
    —Understanding, (with delusions, delirium etc.)
    —Memory

- **Strange, Rare and Peculiar**
  These may occur among mentals, Generals or Particulars and must therefore be of varying importance and rank.
- **Physical**
  —Sexual Perversion (loves and hates, physical)
  —Perversions referred to the stomach
  —Desires and aversion of food
  —Appetite
  —Thirst, for hot and cold etc.
- **Physical Generals**
  —Relations and reactions to environment
  —Time
  —Heat and Cold
  —Damp and Dry
  —Electricity
  —Oxygen and Carbon dioxide
  —Menstrual Aggr & Amel (before, with and after menstruation)
  —Position, Gravitation
  —Pressure, Motion with train sickness etc.
  —Various food aggravations
- **Character of Discharges**
  —Particulars (relating to a part and not to the whole)
  —Observe that in the MENTALS at the beginning, and in the GENERALS at the end, and in all the intermediate sections from cover to cover the same arrangement holds.

  First: Time
  Next: Conditions in alphabetical succession
  then when it is a question of pain

Locality, Character, Extension

Mental: Take a mental symptom from the first section of the Repertory, say "Anxiety"

Anxiety

First – Time

    Morning

    Afternoon

    Night

    At some special hour

Next condtions under which anxiety has been observed in their alphabetical succession.

- **General**

Now turn to the last section Generalities—Here we find agg, amel and reactions of the patients as a whole to physical environment, here precisely the same arrangement is again found.

First – Time

    Morning

    Noon

    Night

    At a particular hour

Among these general agg at the end of the book we find such conditions as Better and Worse.

Pain in general

    —Its onset, gradual or sudden

    —Its disappearance in same ways

    —Its character: burning, pressing, cutting etc.

    —Its direction: up, down, in, out, across, etc.

    —In all, down through the smallest sub-sections, the same order obtains.

- **Uses of Kent's repertory**

  Apart from the use as outlined above we can use this repertory for particular rubrics also. This aspect is usually not known. Select any of the marked symptom/complaint of the patient, you can look for this and compare the remedies shown to select the most applicable for your patient.

  For example: I had a patient whose main complaint was vertigo, it was worse lying on right side. I looked up the Vertigo chapter and found the following entry: **Vertigo, lying right side agg: mur-ac.** I prescribed Muriatic acid which gave complete relief.

  In order to get a good idea of the palcement of various rubrics in Kent's repertory it is recommended to look for the following rubrics:

  1. Sensation of being headless
  2. Hungry after eating
  3. Always washing his hand
  4. Pain above root of the nose
  5. Repeats the question first before answering
  6. Babbling
  7. Speaks in foreign language
  8. Hesitates
  9. Regretful
  10. Picks at the bed clothes
  11. Must restrain himself to prevent doing himself injury
  12. Lazy
  13. Never speaks the truth
  14. Broken bones slow to heal
  15. Cannot hear human voice

An Overview of Repertories for PG Students

16. Heat and cold aggravate
17. On attempting to swallow liquids they come out through the nose
18. Burning sensation in eyes
19. Eyelids remain open in sleep
20. Cannot open the eye lids
21. Brain feels loose
22. Coldness of joints in the morning
23. Swelling like a walnut in left male mammae
24. Bruised feeling in gluteal region
25. Faints in a closed room
26. Itching skin amel by vomiting
27. Pulling pain in back
28. Carbuncle in nape of neck
29. Lacks courage
30. Does not like to bring objects near eyes
31. Sciatica alternating with cough
32. Bed feels hard
33. Cannot bear fingers touching each other
34. Drops things
35. Not well since some illness
36. Abuse of iron aggravates
37. Lips cracked
38. Omits letters in writing
39. Says hot for cold
40. Sexual fancies
41. Does not remember well known streets
42. Malingering
43. Hopeless of recovery

44. Addicted to alcohol
45. Boredom
46. Refuses to eat
47. Making faces
48. •Wringling hands
49. Curious to know
50. Pulls his hair
51. Optimistic
52. Aversion to her child
53. Does the opposite of what he is told
54. Urging for flatus but passes stool instead
55. Objects look inverted
56. Objects look far away
57. Cough ends in sneezing
58. Patient had hemorrhoidal flow suppressed, now has bleeding from lungs
59. One cheek hot the other cold
60. Believes all she says is a lie
61. Dreams of falling
62. Unilateral perspiration
63. Sight of food causes nausea
64. Dreams of falling
65. Unilateral perspiration
66. Sight of food causes nausea
67. Feels he will get diarrhea
68. Time passes too slowly
69. Sweat all over excepting the head
70. Desire to loosen clothing after a meal
71. Sleep walking

72. Cannot weep although sad
73. Frowning
74. Old rags seem as fine as silk
75. Lusiness
76. Urticaria
77. Abscess of glands
78. Sweating gives no relief
79. Choking
80. Child refuses mother's milk
81. Leucorrheal discharge itching
82. Paraphimosis
83. Handles the genitals
84. Erections failing during intercourse
85. Effects of suppressed sex desire
86. Breathing stopped
87. Asphyxia
88. Food goes into larynx when swallowing
89. Sunstroke
90. Edema of glabella
91. Cannot hold up head
92. Disgusted with life
93. Rapid breathing
94. Will not tolerate opposition
95. Body fat with thin legs
96. Wants to die
97. Objects seem to come near and recede
98. Stool soft but difficult
99. Despair from abdominal pain
100. No weakness in spite of diarrhea

101. Stool escapes on laughing
102. Involuntary urination and stool
103. Vomiting with purging
104. Child passes urine and continues to sleep
105. Must urinate 5 or 6 times to empty bladder
106. Cannot urinate in presence of people
107. Addison's disease
108. Stumbles when walking
109. Worries
110. Sexual minded
111. Missing steps when descending
112. Fibroids in uterus
113. Throbbing in head
114. Breath sounds like sawing
115. Cough due to roughness in larynx
116. Doubtful
117. Stool slips back in rectum
118. Worms in stool
119. Daring
120. Cutting pain in ureters
121. Hard testes
122. Fear of water
123. Seeks solitude to do masturbation
124. Itching between thighs
125. Humorous
126. Sexual desire lost in female
127. Uterus retroverted
128. Aphonia
129. Coldness of nipple

130. Unequal breathing
131. Becomes unconscious with cough
132. Cannot expectorate
133. Bloody water oozes from nipple
134. Flushes of heat in spine
135. Black spots in hand
136. Palpitation on swallowing
137. Lordosis
138. Child will sleep only if rocked
139. Car sickness
140. Bubo
141. Forgets names
142. Keloids
143. Eruptions in axillae
144. Excoriation of the perineum
145. Thinks he is persecuted
146. Rocking amel
147. Hungry after eating
148. On laughing urine escapes
149. When coughing always cough twice
150. Sensation of drops of cold water falling from heart
151. Emaciation of neck
152. Sciatic pain aggravated laughing
153. Sensation of paralysis of thumb
154. Chill in upper part of the body
155. Mental depression
156. Asthma
157. Changes mind frequently
158. Symptoms agg. while sweating

159. Sea air agg.
160. Felt as if caged with wires
161. Very talkative during chill
162. Sensation of isolation
163. Cannot make up his mind what to do
164. Emaciation with enormous appetite
165. Euphoria
166. Uurging for stools but passes flatus only
167. Right sided hemiplegia
168. Fear felt in chest
169. Snoring
170. Sensation of cold needles on the skin
171. Carbuncle
172. Feels agg. while seating
173. Feverishness in upper part of the body
174. Feels sleepy during fever
175. Chill comes later every day
176. Trachoma
177. Ptosis of eyelids
178. Pain in head as if hair is pulled
179. While reading letters run together
180. Sensation as if breath came from the ear
181. His own voice seems loud to him
182. Flapping of alae nasi
183. Bad smell of feet without
184. Chill from residing at seashore
185. Chill every 7th day
186. Tenderness of the sternum
187. Difficulty in breathing in diseased conditions of distant

An Overview of Repertories for PG Students 21

            part
188. Tickling in throat pit
189. Orgasm wanting in females
190. Teeth look yellow
191. Ranula
192. Feels like washing face in cold water
193. Dacrocystitis
194. Everything looks golden to the eyes
195. Emptiness in ear
196. Things look absurd
197. Sobbing
198. Dislikes to wear a hat
199. Female patient says "I have aversion to women"
200. Bites the cheek when chewing
201. Pallor of the lips
202. Torticollis
203. Burning in parotid gland
204. Deaf but hears better in noise
205. Desires to drink though he is not thirsty
206. Stools remain long in the rectum
207. Can pass urine only when standing
208. Desire for light

iv. **Synthetic Repertory**

The first edition appeared in 1897. To keep the repertory up-to-date by preserving symptoms and drugs not listed in Kent's Repertory and include their confirmation by cures as well as to make available the primary and repeated proving of younger authors, the Synthetic Repertory (three volumes) containing only general symptoms by Horst Barthel and Will Klunker was published in 1973. It contains

1594 drugs.

Volume I: Psychic Symptoms by Dr. med. Horst Barthel.
Volume II: General Symptoms by Dr. med. Horst Barthel.
Volume III: Sleep, Dreams and Sexuality by Dr. med. Will Klunker.

Others involved in this work are:
- Dr. P. Schmidt of Geneva.
- Dr. Roger Schmidt and Alain Naude of San Francisco.
- Dr. med. Jacques Baur of Lyon.

v. **Kent's Comparative Repertory of the Homeopathic Materia Medica:** Guy Kokelenberg and Rene Dockx.

vi. **Synthesis (Repertorium Homeopathicum Syntheticum):** By Frederik Schroyens in 1993. It is an enlarged Kent's Repertory linked to homeopathic software RADAR based on the sixth edition of Kent's Repertory in totol.

vii. **Complete Repertory:** By Roger Van Zandvoort. Published in 1996.

viii. **Millenium Repertory:** By Roger Van Zandvoort. Published in 1999.

ix. **Thematic Repertory:** By J. A. Mirrili. Published in 1995.

3. **Other Repertories Which Have No Philosophical Basis**

   i. **Alphabetical Repertory**
      - Glazor's first Alphabetical Pocket Repertory at Leipzig in 1833.
      - Clotar Muller – Systematic Alphabetical Repertory in 1848.
      - Bryant – An Alphabetical Repertory in 1851.
      - Phatak's Repertory in 1963; second edition in 1977.

- Homeopathic Medical Repertory (a modern alphabetical repertory) by Robin Murphy, in March 1993. The 2nd edition containing 70 chapters was published in 1997. This repertory has become very popular.

ii. **Concordance Repertory**
- The Concordance repertory of the Materia Medica by William D. Gentry (6 volumes) in 1890.
- Repertory of Hering's Guiding Symptoms by C.B. Knerr in 1896.

iii. **Clinical Repertories**
- Oscar E Boericke's Clinical Repertory appended to handbook of Homeopathic Materia Medica by Dr. William Boericke in 1927.
- A Clinical Repertory to the Dictionary of Materia Medica by Dr. J.H. Clarke.
- Causations by Bhardwaj.
- Times of Remedies by Boger.
- Bell's Diarrhea.
- H.C. Allen's Fevers and others as pointed out earlier.

iv. **Card Repertories**
- W. Guernsey's.
- Boger's.
- Field's.
- Sankaran's (420 cards) (292 remedies) in 1959.
- The Kishore Cards in 1959 and others as pointed out earlier.
- Broussalian Card Repertory in 1969 with 640 remedies and 1861 cases.

v. **Mechanically Aided Repertory**
- Dr. Patel's Autovisual Homeopathic Repertory.
- Dr. Patel's Autovisual Miasmatic Repertory.

vi. Computerized Repertories
- The Lamnia Homeopathic Repertory Analysis System (Australia): It lists 14700 symptoms of Kent's Repertory. It was the first computerized repertory, made probably in the year 1976 or 1977.
- Doctor Georges Broussalian made a repertory containing 10,000 rubrics of Kent's Repertory in 1979. It was named after Hahnemann's second wife as *Le Repertoire De Kent "Melanie"*.
- Mac Repertory by David Warkentin of USA.
- RADAR by Frederik Schroyens of Belgium.
- Hompath by Dr. Jawahar J. Shah of India, Classic 8 version in 2002.
- Kentian by Dr. R P Patel from Sai Homoeopathic Book Corporation, Vadodara.
- HRS developed by CIRA (Centre for Informatics Research and Advancement).
- Polychresta.
- CARA by Dr. Witko.
- Micropath by Micro Therapeutics Ltd., England.
- Homeorep-Boenninghausen's Technique by Dr. Robert Bacheleric, France.
- The Profile by D.J. Vidlard, France.
- The Samuel by The Co-operative Association Holland.
- Stimulare Qu-bit Homeo Technology Bangalore, India.
- Kenbo by Dr. Tarkareshwar Jain, Jaipur, India.
- Mercurius by AEON Group Ltd., Slovakia.
- ISIS by ISIS Inspirational software.
- Organon –96 by Dr. Dixit of ICR Mumbai

Details of Some Lesser Known and Latest Repertories

BOENNINGHAUSEN'S REPERTORIES

Boenninghausen accepted the following fundamentals as proposed by Hahnemann:

— Nothing can be known of a disease except through symptoms.
— It is the patient who is ill and not his parts or organs.
— Symptoms are the only unfailing guide to the selection of the remedy.
— Peculiar, characteristic, individualizing symptoms, as against the common symptoms denote the similar remedy. The remedy can hardly ever be indicated by a single symptom however peculiar it may be.

He proposed four components of Complete Symptom as Location, Sensation, Modality and Concomitant.

He comprehended the difficulties encountered in securing a complete picture of the case (lack of observation existed in provers as existed in patients). He suggested that incomplete symptoms could be reliably completed by analogy. It implies that missing components of a symptom could be completed by analogy.

1. Plan of Boenninghausen's Therapeutic Pocket Book

In this repertory, 342 remedies are included. It is divided into seven parts:

 i. Mind and intellect
 ii. Parts of the body and organs
 iii. Sensation and complaints
   - In general.
   - Of glands.

- Of bones.
- Of skin.

iv. Sleep and Dreams

v. Fever
   - Circulation of blood.
   - Cold stage.
   - Coldness.
   - Heat.
   - Perspiration.
   - Compound fevers.
   - Concomitant complaints.

vi. Alterations of the state of health
   - Aggravations according to time.
   - Aggravations according to situations and circumstances.
   - Amelioration by positions and circumstances.

vii. Relationship of remedies

2. Details of Chapters

i. **Mind and Intellect**

There are very few rubrics (pages 17-23), as it was not his intention to reflect the picture of the whole man through his mental reactions. It was not an oversight as is usually thought. He also realised the difficulty in collecting the mental symptom.

Some examples:

Amativeness.

Avarice.

Boldness.

Gentleness.

An Overview of Repertories for PG Students

Haughtiness.
Mischieviousness.
Mistrust.
Seriousness.
Abusive, scolding, railing etc.
Amorous, amative, lascivious, lewd.
Affectionate.
Agitated.
Ambitious.
Anxiety, agony.
Avarice, covetous.
Aversion to school.
Bad part, takes everything in, easily offended.
Blissful feeling.
Intellect.
Befogged.
Comprehension difficult.
Comprehension easy.
Ecstacy.
Imbecility.
Insanity.
Memory active.
Memory lost.

17 rubrics are devoted to emotional excitement under section Aggravations. Examples are:

Anger, vexation, etc. agg.
Anxiety with agg.
Faultfinding.

Fright, shock with agg.

Indignation with agg.

Silent grief, suppressed, etc.

Violence, with agg.

Contradiction.

Fright [anxiety, fear].

Grief and sorrow, or care agg.

Homesickness.

Jealousy agg.

Joy excessive, agg.

Love unhappy, agg.

Mortification, chagrin, etc. agg.

Reproaches, agg.

Rudeness of others agg.

Sympathy agg.

Wrath, agg.

ii. **Parts of the Body and Organs**

Head-eyes-vision-ears-hearing-nose-smell-face-location of sensation-teeth-gums-mouth-throat-mouth and fauces-hunger and thirst (including aversions and desires)-taste-eructation-nausea and vomiting-internal abdomen-external abdomen-abdomen-hypochondria-abdominal rings-flatulence-stool-urinary organs-urine-micturition-sexual organs-menstruation-leucorrhea-respiration-cough-air passages-external throat and neck-neck and nape of neck-chest-back-upper extremities-lower extremities.

iii **Sensations and Complaints**

Alphabetical arrangement of subjective and objective symptoms.

- In general 54 pages.
- Of glands 4 pages.
  Air passing through, sensation of –spong; atrophy-boring-like knotted cords-suppuration-tearing-cancerous–spong.
- Of bones 3.5 pages.
  Absence of marrow, sensation of-lyc. band sensation of – tension-ulcerative pain.
- Of skin 34 pages.
  Adherent – wrinkled.

Boenninghausen succeeded in condensing the cumbersome features of a repertory and made it comprehensive.

iii Sleep and Dreams

- **Some examples of rubrics of sleep:**

  Yawning
  Without sleepiness
  With stretching
  Yawning ineffectual
  Spasmodic
  Falling asleep late
  Impossible after waking once
  Prevented by various symptoms
  Waking in distress
  Early
  Waking frequently at night
  Late
  Position in sleep
  Lies on abdomen
  Symptoms causing sleeplessness

- **Some examples of dreems** [Dreams in general]
  anxious, anxious of animals
  of battle
  of the dead
  of difficulties
  of falling
  of fire – of ghosts – of bad luck
  of quarrels – of shooting – of sickness
  of thieves-of thunder-of water-
  confused
  of sick people
  of vermin
  of vivid, etc.

v. **Fever**

- Circulation of blood
  Anemia – congestion-pulse
  Abnormal-full-hard
  Imperceptible-slow-small-soft-tremulous, etc.
- Cold stage – chilliness in general – in certain parts.
- Coldness.
- Heat.
- Perspiration.
- Compound fevers.
- Concomitant complaints.

vi. **Alterations in the State of Health**

- Aggravations according to time.
- Aggravations according to situations and circumstances.
- Amelioration by positions and circumstances comparatively small.

Patients report aggravations much more than ameliorations as they are more noticeable.

vii. **Relationship of Remedies**

This last chapter has relationships of remedies for which Boenninghausen is greatly remembered and is used for making the second prescription.

- **Boenninghausen's Concordances**

In the year 1832, Boenninghausen published a work named —**Repertory of the Antipsoric Medicines**. In 1835, he published his—**Repertory of the Medicines which are not Antipsorics**. In 1836, his next work—**An Attempt at Showing the Relative Kinship of Homoepathic Medicines** was published. Actually, this last named work was about the relationship of various homoeopatic medicines. Ultimately, all these books were combined and the great masterpiece—**Therapeutic Pocket Book** appeared in the year 1846.

In the preface of **Therpeutic Pocket Book**, Boenninghausen speaks of his publishing in 1836 the work on relationship of remedies which he later on found to contain a number of errors and omissions, and which he then discarded. Later on, he corrected the work and in the earlier editions of his **Therapeutic Pocket Book**, he incorporated this work as the last chapter and named— *concordance of remedies*. But, when Dr. T.F. Allen edited this work, he changed the name of the chapter as *Relationships of remedies*.

There has always been much speculations regarding the proper method of using Boenninghausen's concordances. While Boenninghausen gave suggestion in the preface of **Therapeutic Pocket Book** for the use of the concordances, yet he did not give full directions.

Consequently, as the suggestions are scanty, they have been overlooked and so the use of concordances has been neglected.

Boenninghausen tells us in his preface something of his method of gathering data; how he kept notes for years on various symptoms, the relationship to each other, and the relationship of remedies to symptom groups. From this accumulated date he devised his **Therapeutic Pocket Book**. With this background we can not believe that any part of the book would be for merely causal use.

- **Utilities**

In speaking of these concordances in the preface. Boenninghausen says "............. this concordance has been of extreme importance, not only for recognition of the genius of the remedy, but also for testing and making sure of its choice, and for judging of the sequence of the various remedies, especially in chronic diseases".

Thus, there are three applications of concordances:

—**Recognition of the genius of remedy:** Boenninghausen puts it, that in studying the materia medica the concordances were of decided importance to him. The basis of such study is the help afforded by the concordance in comparing the remedies. Even Kent recognized it in article—**How to use Boenninghausen's concordances** – "......*If I would take Aconite and desire to study the remedy, I look over this concordances*". Certainly, one way, and perhaps, the most satisfactory way to study the materia medica is by comparison.

—**Greater certainty in selection of remedy:** After a comparative study of materia medica, we can make a logical inference about the remedy which most closely corresponds with a case to be treated.

—**Judgment of sequence of various remedies:** The sequence of the remedies is the most important of the three uses of the concordance. The concordances are to be used to find out the 'next remedy' or the second prescription. The almost always satisfactory result obtained in indicating the remedy to follow is due to the wonderfully accurate and compreshensive manner in which these concordances are compiled.

- **Construction**

The concordance chapter is divided into sections, each section being devoted to a remedy, in alphabetical order. Each of this remedy – sections is subdivided into several rubrics with list of medicines in different grades. In this chapter we find the rubrics are not particularized as symptoms but are generalized symptom groups. These rubrics are arranged in each remedy-sections in the following order–

Mind

Localities

Sensations

Glands

Bones

Skin

Sleep and Dreams

Blood, circulation and fever

Aggravations: Time and circumstances

Other remedies

Antidotes

Injurious

Each remedy partakes to some extent in the domain of every other remedy. These common features are described by

Boenninghausen as *points of contant*. Therefore in concordance chapter, we find in each remedy-sections, these *points of contants* (i.e. rubrics) with different remedies starting from **Mind** upto **Aggravations: Time and circumstances**. There may be some symptoms which can not be grouped under these regular rubrics, then one should consider the rubric – **Other remedies**. Of the other two rubrics – **Antidotes** and **Injurious**, which occasionally appear – they are self-explanatory by their names.

To find out the second prescription we may use the following chart –

Medicines	Mind	Localities	Sensations	Glands	Bones	Skin	Sleep and Dreams	Blood, Circulation & Fever	Aggravation: Time & Circumstances	Other Remedies	Total

—First of all, open the section of the medicine which is the first prescription. That means, if the first prescription is Aconite, then to work out the second prescription consult the section of Aconite from Boenninghausen's concordance chapter.

—Consider the chief symptom of the case and select the first rubric accordingly. Thus, if it be mental symptom **Mind** is used first, or if the part (be elsewhere in the body) then the rubric – **Localities** is taken first, if it be a pain, choose the rubric **Sensations** as the first rubric, and so on.

—Note down names of all medicines present in the chosen first rubric in the medicine column of the chart. Then note down the ranks (1, 2, 3, 4, or 5) of these medicines in that chosen rubric column.

—Then record the ranks of the medicines present in other rubrics of the same section in corresponding rubric columns in the chart by considering only those medicines which appear in the first rubric.

—Then in the total column of each medicine write down the summations of the ranks and total matching.

—Then consider only those drugs which are shown higher rankings and more matching and compare them with the patients's symptomatology and finally come to a conclusion of the second prescriptions. But if this medicine is present in **Antidote** or **Injurious** rubric, discard it and consider the next similar medicine as second prescription.

- **Conclusion**

Thus from what has been detailed so far, we may conclude that Boenninghausen's concordance may be used in several ways with excellent results; particularly it is of utmost value in selecting the second prescription which it does with accuracy and with minimum expenditure of time and labour.

BOGER BOENNINGHAUSEN REPERTORY - 1905

This is an updated edition of Boenninghausen's Therapeutic Pocket Book by C.M. Boger. The base of BBCR is Therapeutic Pocket Book, which explained below:

1. **Plan and Construction**

   i. **Mind and Intellect, including Sensorium and Vertigo** from pages 191-250.

ii. **Locations i.e., Sensation and Complaints** experienced in different locations i.e., anatomical parts of the body and organs according to the Hahnemannian schema, viz., Head (250-308); Eyes (309-348); Ears (348-364); Nose (365-390); Face (390-416); Teeth (416-440); Mouth (441-472); Appetite/Thirst, etc. (472-499); Nausea and Vomiting (500-513); Stomach and Hypochondria (514-544); Abdomen; Inguinal and Pubic Region (544-571); Flatulence, Stool and Anus (572-575); Urine and Urinary Organs (576-618); Genitalia, Male and Female (645-668); Sexual Impulse (669-674); Menstruation (675-689); Respiration (690-705); Cough and Expectoration (705-733); Larynx and Trachea (734-738); Voice (738-742); Neck and External Throat (743-748); Nape (748-752); Chest (753-772); Heart and Region of Heart (773-784); Back, Scapular, Dorsal, Lumbar, etc. (784-804) Upper Extremities (805-842); Lower Extremities (843-881).

iii. **Sensations and Complaints in General** (881-936); of Glands (937-940); of Bones (940-944); of Skin and Exterior body (944-979).

iv. **Sleep and Dreams** (980-1002).

v. **Fever** – Pathological types (1002-1005); Blood (1005-1006); Palpitation, Heart beat; Pulse (1006-1020); Fever in general (1047-1076); Sweat (1076-1098); Compound fever (1099-1102).

vi. **Conditions of Aggravation and Amelioration in General**– of Time (1103-1104); of Situations, Positions, Circumstances, etc. (1105-1153).

vii. **Concordances (Relationship of Remedies)** (1154-1231)

2. Advantages Over Kent's Repertory

Each physician who attempts to use Kent's Repertory, requires knowledge of evaluation of symptoms into general, particular and common symptoms and any error in the process of evaluation may throw away the indicated drug out of repertorial analysis. One has to be very sure as to the exact interpretation of mental symptoms and their value in the repertorization. It is a fact that in practice, it is not always possible to carry out Kentian evaluation in each case and many a time forceful extraction of generals, especially mental generals in one-sided chronic cases gives a poor response to repertory based prescription.

In cases seen in practice, it is very easy to complete four elements of each symptom according to Boger Boenninghausen's concept of totality of complete symptoms as it does not require any sophisticated understanding of evaluation of symptoms. One has to just separate location, sensation, modality and concomitants. Each component of the complete symptom can be a characteristic symptom of a drug or a patient e.g.:

Left sided complaints	–	*Lachesis*
Right sided complaints	–	*Lycopodium*
Right forehead	–	*Silicea, Sanguinaria*
Left forehead	–	*Spigelia*
Liver	–	*Chelidonium*
Pancreas	–	*Iris versicolor*
Spleen	–	*Ceanothus*

The list is very long and similar observations can be made as regards characteristic sensations (*stinging of Apis, burning of Cantharis and Arsenicum album*), modalities, concomitants (*thirstlessness with dryness of mouth of Pulsatilla*) of drugs. In our day to day materia medica based prescribing of acute cases, we are utilizing Boenninghausen's concept of evaluation of symptoms. The suitability, applicability and value of Boger Boenninghausen's Repertory for each case is much more than any other repertory available to us. It may be mentioned that Kent used Boenninghausen's repertory for 20 years.

3. Diagnositic/Clinical-Rubrics in BBCR

Abcess	Chordee
Atheroma	Corns
Acne	Cretinism
Apthae	Cough
Ascitis	Convulsions
Asphyxia	Croup
Asthma	Cardalgia
Aneurysm	Colic
Apoplexy	Condylomata
Anemia	Chancre
Amenorrhea	Chancroid
Acne comedo	Cysts
Anorexia	Cheyne-stokes respiration
Anthrophobia	Carphology
Acetoneuria	Cancerous Cachexia
Abortion	Canpulency
Angina Pectoris	Chilbains
Atrophy	Cicatrices
Anthrax	Chloasmae
Bronchitis	Diptheria
Boils	Diarrhea
Cataract	Dysentery
Cancer	Diuresis
Cirrhosis	Dyspnea
Calculi	Dropsy
Carbuncle	Dyscrasia

Encephalitis	Gleet
Erysipelas	Ganglion
Ecchymoses	Hydrocephalus
Epithelioma	Hypopion
Epilepsy	Herpes
Epistaxis	Hemiopia
Eczema	Hemorrhoids
Erythema	Hydronephrosis
Ebullition	Hydrocele
Eclampsia	Hydrothorax
Exctosis	Hemophilia
Epithelioma	Hydrophobia
Erysipelas	Hemorrhage
Excreascences	Hypochondriacs
Exanthematous typhus	Hernia
Fistula	Hysteria
Fissure	Hypertrophy
Fungoid growths	Hyperesthesia
Fracture	Hectic fever
Glaucoma	Helminthiasis
Gangrene	Impotency
Goitre	Inflammation acute
Gout	Influenza
Gonorrhea	Induration
Gastralgia	Intussusception
Gall stone	Ischuria
Gravel	Impetigo

Intermittent fever	Oedema
Jaundice	Oesophagitis
Kyphosis	Oxaluria
Keloid	Onanism
Lichen	Osteomyelitis
Lupus	Pterigium
Leucorrhea	Ptosis
Lochia	Polyp
Lumbago	Periostitis
Lethargy	Phimosis
Meningitis	Prolapsus
Migraine	Priapism
Myopia	Pthysis
Myoma	Pleurodynia
Miliaria	Pneumonia
Myelitis	Paralysis agitans
Mentagra	Plague
Miliaria	Polypi
Malaria	Phagadena
Measles	Paraplegia
Metastasis	Photophobia
Malaise	Polyuria
Marasmus	Presbyopia
Neuralgia	Pustules
Necrosis	Pimples
Nevus	Peritonitis
Opisthotonus	Pneumatocele

Phosphaturia
Phimosis
Pudendal-abcess
Phlegmasia dolens
Rickets
Risus Sardonicus
Retained placenta
Rheumatism
Sarcoma
Strabismus
Styes
Stomatitis
Subinvolution
Satyriasis
Spina bifida
Sciatica
Small pox
Scurvy
Syphillis
Trichiasis

Trachoma
Tumor
Tuberculosis
Tetanic
Tinia
Tarter
Tympanitis
Typhoid fever
Uraemia
Ulcers
Varicosity
Voluvlus
Vesicles
Varicocele
Varicella
Warts
Whooping cough
Yellow fever
Zoster (Zona)

4. Some Important Rubrics in the BBCR

Symptoms	Rubrics
Complaints after Vaccination	Agg & Amel in general – vaccination agg. (1148)
Cannot bear to stay in a close room	Agg & Amel in general – room in the agg. (1138)
	Agg & Amel in general – Vaulted Places (1148)
Homesickness	Mind – homesickness (203)
	Agg & Amel in general – Emotion homesickness (1116)
Risus saradonicus	Face – Risus sardonicus (400)
	Mind – laughter – Sardonic (209)
	Sens & complaint – tetanic or symptoms, tetanic flexor or cramps (930)
Diabetes mellitus	Urine – Saccharine (622)
Likes to eat pickles	Appetite – desire for pickles (477)
Person denies being sick	Sens & complaint in general – well, feeling – sense of well being (denies of being sick); (936)
Travelling sickness	Agg & Amel in general – driving or riding in carriage agg. (1114)

An Overview of Repertories for PG Students

	Nausea & Vomiting – Agg – driving (507)
	Vertigo – agg driving (242)
Urinary Calculi	Urinary organs – Kidney's calculi (638)
Taste of Spoiled fat	Taste – Putrid meat of (486)
	Taste – Rancid – (486)
	Taste – Spoiled – (488)
Does not like tobacco product	Appetite – Aversion to tobacco (smoke) (475)
Complaints of drunkards	Stomach & epigastrium – Agg whisky (530), wine
	Abodomen – Agg – whisky abuse of (565)
	Agg & Amel in general – drunkards (1114)
Uric acid diathesis	Agg & Amel in general – uric acid diathesis (1148)
Aneurysms	Fever – Circulation – Blood vessel varicose (1007)
	chest – heart region of Aneurysm (773)
Hypertrophical Tonsil enlarge, swollen	Mouth – Throat & Gullet – Tonsil – hypertrophy (457)
Concussion of brain	Head internal – concussion of brain after (283)
Blenorrhea	Eyes – Blenorrhea (310)
Groaning	Mind – groaning (moaning) (203)
Imparied digestion (d)* pregnancy	Stomach & epigastrium Agg – pregnancy (d) (529)

	Stomach – Digestion impaired – (d) Pregnancy (516)
Complaints (a)* shellfish	Agg & Amel in general – food & drinks shellfish agg. (1122) Agg & Amel in general – food & drinks oyster agg (1121)
Gall stones	Hypochondria – gall stone & colic (536) gall bladder inflammed (536)
Gastric complaint after ice cream	Stomach & epigastrium – Agg ices frozen (528)
Dropsy	Sens & complaint in general – drospy, edema of external parts (894) Lower extremeties – dropsy (853) Upper extremeties – dropsy (816)
Volvulus	Abdomen – Volvulus (559)
Small-pox	Skin & exterior body – Smallpox – variola (9.65)
Herpes	Skin & exterior body – Tetters (including herpes and eczema) (968)
Shingles	Skin & extr. body – zoster (Zona) (979)
Chicken pox	Skin & exterior body – variolla (976)

Urticaria	Skin & exterior body – erruption – urticarious (nettle rash) (953)
Nocturnal enuresis	Urine – micturation – urination night in bed (bed wetting) (627)
Feels as if in a dream (error of locality)	Mind – Bewildered strange (194) Mind – dream as in a (199)
Varicocele	Genitalia – testis – varicocele (645)
Climatic Migraine	Head internal – (Migraine) Head aggravation – climatic (282)
Giddiness with double vision	Vertigo – Realing staggering, giddy (240) Vertigo – diplopia with (248)
Starchy food	Agg & Amel in general – food drinks – farinaceous (1122)
Does not like washing	Agg & Amel in general – water & washing agg (1151)
Scabies	Skin & exterior body – itch (scabies) (956)
Nevus	Skin & exterior body – Nevus maternus (963)
Inability to sleep though sleepy	Sleep – Sleeplessness although sleepy (995) Sleep – Sleepiness sleep with inability to (986)
Intolerance of breast milk	Agg & Amel in general – food & drinks milk agg. of mother's agg. (1121)

Eructation odour of Sulphur	Eructation – Eggs, like bad (or sulphuretted hydrogen) (491)
Stammering in old age	Voice & speech – stammering (741)
	Voice & speech – Senility, Agg. (742)
Quotidian fever	Fever – Pathological types Intermittent – quotidian (1003)
Lumbricoids	Stool – worms lumbricoides with (592)
Jesting	Mind – Tedium ennui (219)
Quartan fever	Fever – Pathological type – Intermittent quartan (1004)
Sea sickness	Agg & Amel in general ship board on agg (1140)
	Agg & Amel in general sea at agg (1139)
	Vertigo – agg ship board on (245)
Scurvy	Sens & Complaint in general – Scurvy, scrobutic symptoms (918)
Sinuses	Nose – internal sinuses (365)
Desire to be alone	Mind – solitude love of (217)
	Mind – comprany – Averse to (195)
	Agg & Amel in general – Alone desires solitude (1106)
	Agg & Amel in general – Society – company of people agg (1142)

Gall-Bladder	Hypochondria – Gall bladder (536)
Ganglion (bursae)	Bone – Ganglion (bursae) (941)
Fracture	Bones – Fracture (941)
Rachitis	Bone – Curvature, curve, deformaed (941)
Puberty youth	Sens & compl in general – Puberty youth (915)
Complaints occur in one spot	Sens & complaint in general – spots, sensations occur in (923)
Hectic fever	Fever – pathological type – Intermittent Tertian (1004)
Asphyxia	Sens & complaint in general – Asphyxia (883) Respiration – Asphyxia (neonatorum) (690)
Nape	Neck & external throat – Nape (748)
Complaints (during) micturition	Urine – during urination (631)
Does not like open air	Agg & Amel in general – Air open agg. (1105) Agg & Amel in general – air open agg. (1118)
Missing a meal amel or complaints better by fasting	Abdomen – Amel – fasting (566)
Nipples retracted	Chest – nipples – retracted (772)
Abcess in axilla	Chest – axilla – abscess (767)
Coryza excoriating	Nose – discharge acid (369)

Capriciousness	Mind – changeable (194)
Nursing agg	Agg & Amel in general – Suckling (nursing) the infant agg (1144)
Asthma milleri	Respiration – asthma milleri (691) larynx & trachea – Spasm of cramp (asthma milleri) (737)
Unsocial	Agg & Amel in general – Society company of people agg. (1142)
Lachrymal fistula	Eyes – fistula lachrymal (312)
Eructation alternating with hiccough	Hiccough – Hiccough, erructation alternating with (498)
Pericarditis	Chest – Heart region of Pericardium (772)
Chest – Heart region of Inflammation of (774)
Varicose vein	Fever – circulation – Blood vessel – varicose veins especially (1007)
Periodicity of symptom	Agg & Amel in general – Periodically (1135)
Muscle does not respond to will	Mind – Muscles do not respond to will (212)
Uterine spasms	Sens & complaint in general – spasms uterine (923)
Agg in open air	Sens & complaint in general – air averse to open (881)

Infants affection of	Sens & complaint in general – Infants affection of (903)
Loss of vital fluid	Agg & Amel in general – loss of vital fluid (1128)
Acidity	Stomach – acidity – sour stomach (514) Waterbrash & heart burn – heart burn (495) Erructation – Sour, (493)
Herpetic erruption with burning	Skins & exterior body – Tetters-burning (968)
Remedies fail to act	Sens & complaint in general – Medicines, susceptibility, wanting (908)
Infantile jaundice	Sens & Complaint in general – Infants Jaundice (903)
Jaundice	Skin & exterior body – color yellow, jaundice (947)
Headache with increased urination	Head internal – Agg. Urinary, crises, polyuria with (291)
Lumbago during leucorrhea	Menstruration – leucorrhea – Concomitant lumbar pain (690)
Lumbago during pregnancy	Back agg pregnancy (during) (802)
Complaints during pregnancy	Agg & Amel in general, Pregnancy during agg (1135)
Globus hystericus	Mouth Throat & gullet – Globus as of a ball, lump (hystericus) (452)
Diverting the mind amel	Agg & Amel in general, Diverting the mind amel (1113)

Music intolerance of	Agg & Amel in general, Music intolerance of agg (1133)
Aversion to music	Mind Aversion to music (193)
Hemophilia	Sens & complaint in general hemophilia (901)
Prostalic fluid loss of during stool	Sexual impulse – Prostatic fluid loss of, stool during (671)
Cheyne stoke respiration	Respiration – cheyne stokes respirations (691)
Inguinal hernia	Inguinal & Pubic region – Hernia inguinal (573)
Affected parts appear dead	Sens & complaint in general – Dead appearances of affected parts (891)
Complaints caused by punishment	Agg & Amel in general – Punishment, agg (1136)
Pains come & go suddenly	Sens & complaints in general – Sudden, effects, pains coming and going (926)
	Sens & complaint in general – come & go quickly pains go (888)
Senility	Agg & Amel in general Old age, senility, agg in (1134)
Complaints of hard drinkers	Agg & Amel in general drunkards (topers) (1114)
Frozen limbs	Lower extremity – Frozen, as if (855)
Eructation & Hiccough comes alternatively	Hiccough – hiccough, eructation, alternating with (498)

Understands question only when repeated	Mind – Answers – repeats question first (192)
Never speaks the truth	Mind – lies – habitually (210)
Sun agg	Agg & Amel in general – Sun (heat of) in the agg (1144)
Alternating mental & physical symptoms	Mind – Alternating with Physical symptoms (191)
Anthrophobia	Mind – Anthrophobia (192)
Disgust for everything	Mind – Aversion to, disgust, for everything (193)
Tranquility	Calmness, composure, tranquility (194)
Hardness of heart	Mind – Deceit, cunning, Kryptomania (197)
Unsatisfied, wants this or that	Mind – dissatisfied, discontent, wants this then that (198)
Feels that some one else is sick	Mind – Duality seems as if someone else were sick (199)
Confusion of future with the past	Mind – Future confounds the future with the past (202)
Murder	Mind – Homicidal, murder etc. (203)
Hydrophobia	Mind – Hydrophobia (204) Sens & complaint in general – Hydrophobia (902)
Hypochondriasis	Mind – Hypochondriasis (204) Sens & complaint in general hypochordriasis & hysteria (902)
Hysteria	Mind – Hysteria (204)

	Sens & complaint in general – Hypochondriasis & hysteria (902)
Sick feeling	Mind – Illness sense of & sick feeling (205)
	Sens & complaint – Ill sense of being (sick feeling) (902)
	Sens & complaint – unwell indisposed; attacks of being (933)
Hesitation	Mind – Indecision – hesitation (207)
Aversion to work	Mind – Indolence, aversion to work (208)
Madness alternation with symptom of the disposition	Mind – Insanity, alternating with symptoms of the disposition (208)
Lack of interest	Mind interest lack of (208)
Learns late to speak	Mind – learning to speak, late in (210)
Does not like to be looked at	Mind – looked at aversion to being (210)
False perception of spots infront of eyes	Eyes – Vision illusion spots (343)
Epistaxis during diptheria	Nose – Bleeding diptheria during (367)
Complaints appear exactly at the same hour	Condition in general – Periodically, at exactly the same hour – (1104)
Reopening of old wounds	Skin & exterior body – wounds reopening of old (979)

	Cicatrices reopening of old (946)
Missing of every 3rd pulse beat	Fever circulation, Pulse – intermittent losing the 3rd beat (1014)
Apoplexy	Sens & complaint in general, Apoplexy (882)
Chlorosis	Sens & complaint in general – chlorosis (887)
Desire to be carried, in children	Sens & complaint in general – carried desire to be (children) (887)
Upper left and lower right	Sens & complaint in general – side left, upper left & lower right (920)
Infantile diarrhea	Sens & complaint in general - Infants affections of diarrhea (902)
Fontanalles remain open	Sens & complaint in general, Infants affection, fontanalles open (903)
Ophthalimia neonatorum	Sens & complaint in general - Infants affections eyes, ophthalmia etc. (903)
Metastasis	Sens & complaint in general - metastasis (908)
Carphology	Sens & complaint in general - Carphology (886)
Restlessness	Mind - Restlessness (214) Sens & complaints in general - Restlessness, corporal (917)

Somnambulism	Mind - somnambulism (217)
Uremia	Sens & complaint in general - uremia (934)
Learning late to walk	Sens & complaint in general - walk, children learn to, with difficulty (934).
Sociable	Mind - sociable (217)
Desire for open air	Sens & complaint in general – Air to open (881)
Aversion for open air	Sens & complaint in general Air averse to open (881)
Puerperal fever	Genitalia female - childbed - puerperal fever (658) Fever - Pathological type - Puerperal fever (1004)
Wants to escape from the bed	Mind - escape from bed (200)
Children reject the things when offered	Mind - Desires things which are rejected when offered (198)
Bronchial asthma	Respiration - asthma bronchial (690)
Crepitation	Respiration - crepitation (691)
Heart goitre	Chest, heart and region of, goitre heart (774)
Delayed dentition	Teeth - dentition, slow, difficulty (420)
Psoriasis	Skin & exterior body - eruption in general scaly, psoriatic (952)
Parkinsonism	Sens & complaint in general - Paralysis agitans (911)

Discouraged during pregnancy	Mind - despairing, discouraged, Pregnancy during (198)
Helminthiasis	Agg & Amel in general worms, helminthiasis agg (1153)
Running water agg	Agg & Amel in general - water & washing running agg, from hearing or seeing (1151)
Walking on a narrow bridge aggravation	Agg & Amel in general - walking on a narrow bridge agg (1149)
Cervico bracialis	Neck & external throat - Neuralgia, brachialia and cervico brachialis (745)
Goitre	Neck & external throat - Thyroid gland (goitre) (747)
Venous goitre	Neck & external throat - Thyroid, venous goitre (747)
Torticollis	Neck & external throat wry neck, torticollis (748)
Uncertain gait	Lower ext - stumbling, uncertain, gait lower ext - Gait, uncertain, unsteady
Awkward	Lower Ext - Gait, awkward - awkward lower Ext - awkward
Snoring	Respiration - Inspiration, snoring (692) Respiration - snoring (694)

	Sleep - during sleep, snoring (989)
Hydrothorax	Chest - inner hydrothorax (757)
Pleurodynia	Chest inner - Pleurodynia (758) chest external, pleurodynia (766)
Asthenic Pneumonia	Chest inner pneumonia, asthenic type (senile) (759)
Hot Breath	Respiration - Hot breath (692)
Sensation of cold air while inspiration	Respiration - Inspiration, cold air seems (692)
Sensation as if breathing through a sponge	Respiration - Sponge, as if through a (694) Respiration - Wedding or cloth, as if through (695)
Gets a suffocative attack & so must bend the body backward & sit upright	Respiration - suffocative attack must sit upright & bend the body backwards (692)
Difficult resp. sens as if from the whole body is pressed	Respiration - difficult (691) Respiration impeded by - pressed, full sensation as if the body were (698)
Asthma alternating with skin symptoms	Respiration - asthma (690) Resp - aggravation - skin symptom alternating with (702)
Asthma better by sitting straight & bending forward	Respiration - asthma (690) Resp - Amel - sitting upright & bend forward with (704)

An Overview of Repertories for PG Students

Rattling of mucus in throat chest after walking in	Resp - Ratting (mucus) throat in, (693) Resp - agg - walking in open air after (703)
Asthmatic wheezing	Cough - asthmatic, wheezy (705)
Wheezing	Respiration - Tight, wheezing (694)
Violent cough	Cough - forcible, violent, hard (706)
Continous coughing	Cough - Incessant (706)
Violent first cough followed by weaker & weaker cough	Cough -Paroxysms - the first cough the most violent, the succeeding coughs weaker and weaker (706)
Parotid glands swollen, if touched with anything woolen	Cough - excited & agg by - Parotid gland swollen if, touched with anything woolen (714)
Feels as if a foreign body is present on swallowing	Cough - excited or agg by - larynx, foreign body in, as if when swallowing (713) chest inner foreign body in, as of a (757)
Difficulty in breathing	Respiration - Difficult (691) Respiration - Expiration - Difficult (691) Respiration, Tightness of chest (693)

	Respiration, want of breath, recover his breath can't (694)
Hemorrhage	Cough - Expectoration, Hemorrhage (729) Sens & Compl, - Hemorrhages (901) Fever, Blood, Veins (1006)
Hemoptysis	Cough - Expectoration Blood - blood pure hemoptysis (728)
Phthisis of larynx	Larynx & trachea - Phthisis (736)
Talks in the same tone	Voice & speech - Monotonus (740)
Talks in a rough voice after measles	Voice & speech - condition of voice - measles after (742)
Sub maxillary glands	Neck & external throat - glands, cervical (& submaxillary) (744)
Abscess in the pulmonary region	Chest - Inner - Strenum & region of abcess, pulmonary (754)
Pain in the chest radiates from right to left	Chest - Inner - Direction of pain, right to left (756)
Rush of blood to the chest	Chest - Inner - orgasm, rush of blood. (758)
Neglected Pneumonia in senile people	Chest - Inner - Pneumoria asthenic type (senile), prolonged, neglected etc. (759)

Miliary eruption on chest	Chest - external - miliary eruption (765)
Mammae congested with milk with co-existent mental distrubance	Chest - Mammae - congested with milk, with co-existent mental disturbance (769)
Appearance of milk with absence of menses in spinsters	Mammae - Milk appearance of, without child bearing, form suppressed menses (770)
Galactorrhea	Chest - Mammae - Milk, galactorrhea (770)
Hypertrophy of heart	Chest - Heart and Region of - hypertrophy (774)
Opisthotonos	Back - spinal column & vertebrae - opisthotonos & Back proper - dorsal region Back - Bending backward (789) Sens & complaints in general - opisthotonos (911)
Kyphosis	Back - back proper region - Kyphosis (791)
Callosities in hand	Upper - extremities - callosities (H) (811)
One sided (Migraine) – in anemic people	Head - Internal - half of one (Migraine) Head - Internal - agg - Anemia from
Congestion in brain	Head Internal - Congestion - head (259)

Headache gradually & stops suddenly	Head - Internal - Increases gradually & ceases suddenly (285)
Meningitis	Head Internal - Inflammation Meningitis (265)
Encephalitis	Head Internal - Inflammation - encephalitis (265)
Prurigo	Head external - erruption itching (prurigo) (301)
Pityriasis	Head external - erruption scaly branlike (pityriasis) (301)
Plica polonica	Head external - erruption - plica polonica (301) Head external - Plica polonica (305)
Falling of hair in bunches from head	Head external - hair falling out, in bunches, spots etc. (302)
Photophobia	Eyes - Photophobia (315)
Alternate contraction & dilation of pupil	Eyes - Pupil - alternately contracted & dilated (316)
Sand like sensation in eyes	Eyes - Sand, in, as of (317)
Strabismus	Eyes - strabismus (317)
Trichiasis	Eyes - Trichiasis (319)
Apathy	Mind - Indifference - apathy (207)
Despondancy	Mind - Dejection despondancy (197)
Tranius	Mind - Imagination, fancies, fixed ideas (207)

An Overview of Repertories for PG Students   61

Perverse	Mind - headstrong, destinated, defiant, stubborn (203)
Restless	Mind - Indifference, apathy (207)
Chloasma	Genitalia female Organs, pregnancy face, chloasma (662)
Inosmia acute cold	Nose, smell - weak catarrah from (380)
Tuberculosis	Chest Inner - Tuberculosis (763)
	Complaints & Sensation - consumption in general (889)
	Abdomen - Tuberculosis of (558)
	Larynx & trachea - Pthisis (736)
Neuralgia	Chin - mentagra (413)
Taste of spoiled fat	Taste - Rancid (487)
Abdominal complaints due to shell fish	Agg & Amel in general - food & drinks, shell fish (1122)
Sterility	Female organs - Barrenness, sterility (657)
Reopening of old wounds	Skin & Ext body - wounds reopening of old (978)
Febris helodes	Fever - pathological types - Sudoral fever (1004)
Aversion to bathing	Mind - Aversion to bathing (193)

Hydrogenoid constitution	Sensation & Comp - Constitution hydrogenoid (888)
Diarrhea (during) dentition	Sensation & Complaint - Infants affection of dentition with diarrhea (903)
Illusion of crackling, drumming, echoing	Ear-hearing illusion of bellowing (359)
Milk fever (lactation)	Fever Pathological types - milk fever (945)
Perspiration of upper part of body	Sweat partial sweat - upper parts (1079)
Direction of pain cross wise	Sens. Compl- Direction of pain cross wise (892)
Brittle nail	Skin & Ext body - Nail Brittle. (962)
Corpulency – (obesity)	Sens. & Comp. - obesity (911)
Stool has, to be removed mechanically	Constipated - mechanically removed only (584)
Sides of the body diagonal	Sens. & Complaint - side, diagonal, cross ways (920)
Hysterical fainting	Sensorium - fainting hysterical (237)

Selected Rubrics* of Frequent Reference in case of Osteoarthritis and its Associate Complaints

Arthritic pain

Aged, old

Activity, motion amel.

Ascending steps agg.

Awaking when agg.

Back scapular

Back dorsal

Back lumbar

Band, ligature sensation

Bones, aching pain

Boring, piercing

Burrowing, digging pain

Bed in, retiring, amel

Bending affected part agg.

Bent, holding the part agg

Climacteric agg

Cervical vertebra

Condition of agg annel,

Curvature, curve, deformed

Congestion

Constitiution

Consumption in general

Condylese pain in

Co-ordination affected

Crepitating, crackling feeling in joints
Cold in general agg
Caries, bone
Direction of the symptoms
Dead sense of single part
Dancing agg
Descending step agg
Dislocation, sprains agg
Driving agg
Drawing in affected part
Epiphysis
Excoriative pain
Exertion, physical agg
Enlargement sense of
Expanded feeling
Extosis
Exudations
Eating or phagedenic process
Faintness on rising
Feebleness
Flowing like a hot current
Flying Pain
Female, for agg
Feet, motion of agg
Gnawing, eating in, bones
Gritting in joints

Group symptoms appear
Hot water amel
Hard bed sense of
Hardness
Heaviness of ext. part
Heaviness, load like a
Hypersthesia
Hair brushing agg
Holding part together agg
Hip and loin region
Idleness agg
Ileo coecal region
Induration
Increasing & decreasing of pain
Jerking and catching pain in ext. part
Kyphosis
Lumbar region
Lancinating Pain
Lie down, inclined to
Lying in bed-agg
Lightining, electric like pain
Labor, manual agg
Limb, extended
Lifting and overlifting agg
Mollification/softening
Motion absent, Immobhility

Moving pains, muscles in general, stiff
Moon, new agg
Monthly, continues amel
Neck, turning agg
Nape (cervical region)
Needle like pain
Nodes
Neurasthenia, exhaustion
Obesity
Obtuse pain
Occupational disorders, Cramps
Outward pains move
Old age, senility
Periodicity, Intermittent
Painfulness
Phagedaena
Pinching in ext. part
Plethora
Plug a nail in ext. parts
Projection, bone of
Position must change
Puffiness
Pressure in joints
Pulling or drawing down
Piano playing agg
Pain, agg, during
Raising affected part agg

Rest amel
Revelling (night) agg
Rising from seat, when agg
Rubbing message, gentle agg. But hard as amel.
Rending, shattering pain
Running agg.
Radiation pain
Raw pain
Rigidity of muscles
Rheumatism
Rest must
Restlessness of limbs, can't sit
Retraction of soft parts
Rheumatic pain
Rigid feeling
Stiffness
Swelling
Sides
Sycosis
Syphillis
Scrapes in bones
Shooting pain
Sickening pain
Sit, impulse to
Squeezing pain in ext. part
Stabbing pain
Sticking in joints in

Stooped gait

Stunning pain

Stump, pain in, neuralgia of

Support, the body with difficult

Sedentary occupation agg.

Stepping hard agg.

Tension, tightness in general

Transverse pains

Temperature change agg.

Tearing in bones

Upward down movement, pain of

Vitality decreasing

Weakness, muscular, of joint, senile

White, swelling, hydrops articuli

Wind or draft blowing on parts

Wood feelings as if made of

Wave like pain

Walking beginning of agg

KNERR'S REPERTORY

It is an index to Hering's Guiding Symptoms and was prepared by Dr. Calvin B. Knerr.

1. *Plan and Construction*

The order of arrangement or method of classification, followed in the compilation of this repertory is the one inaugurated by Hahnemann, while it was developed, perfected and used by Hering throughout his entire materia medica work viz., the anatomical or regional division into forty eight chapters. It is based on the language of the patient hence, the rubrics are very long but they are very precise.

List of Chapters

(1) Mind and Disposition Sensorium (2) Inner Head (3) Outer Head (4) Eyes (5) Ears (6) Nose (7) Upper Face (8) Lower Face (9) Teeth and Gums (10) Taste and Tongue (11) Inner Mouth (12) Throat (13) Desires, Aversions Appetite, Thirst (14) Eating and Drinking (15) Hiccough, Belching, Nausea and Vomiting (16) Scrobiculum and Stomach (17) Hypochondria (18) Abdomen (19) Stool and Rectum (20) Urinary Organs (21) Male Sexual Organs (22) Female Sexual Organs (23) Pregnancy, Parturition, Lactation (24) Voice Larynx Trachea and Bronchia (25) Respiration (26) Cough and Expectoration (27) Inner Chest and Lungs (28) Heart Pulse and Circulation (29) Outer Chest (30) Neck and Back (31) Upper Limbs (32) Lower Limbs (33) Limbs in General (34) Rest, Position, Motion (35) Nerves (36) Sleep (37) Time (38) Temperature and Weather (39) Fever (40) Attacks, Periodicity (41) Locality and Direction (42) Sensation in General (43) Tissues (44) Touch, Passive Motion, Injuries (45) Skin (46) Stages of Life and Constitution (47) Drug Relationships (48) Index.

Each chapter is alphabetically divided into sections and rubrics without destroying its consistency as a whole. The basic difference of this repertory from *Allen's Symptoms Register* is that it contains symptoms and remedies not only from provings but confirmations also. To represent it, different grades have been used.

I   The lowest a single light line designating an occasionally confirmed symptom.

II   A double light line indicates a symptom more frequently confirmed or it has confirmed only once confirmed strictly in character with the genius of the remedy.

I   A singly heavy line under a drug indicates that a symptom has been verified by cures.

‖ A double heavy line, symptom has been repeatedly verified. These degree marks tally with the four styles of type used by Boenninghausen.

π represents symptoms observed on the sick only.

t represents toxicological symptoms.

This Concordance Repertory is one of the few repertories where symptoms have been placed unbroken by preserving the original words/expressions so that they retain the most delicate shades of meaning to maintain individuality which is very vital in the selection of the simillimum. Generalization has the drawback of destroying the fine delicacy of symptoms as has been with Boenninghausen repertories and to some extent with Kent's Repertory. Let us take example of the mental symptom –Forgetful. Knerr has listed first, all the remedies which have forgetfulness in general followed by smaller rubrics which have special association with a particular circumstance or condition or are related to a specific time frame in an alphabetical order. This arrangement though systematic and good is impractical in the repertorization process. Therefore, this repertory though useful, has been rarely used by the profession.

In comparison to Kent's Repertory, rubric placing is more appropriate in Knerr's Repertory e.g., Jaundice has been placed under the section Liver; Gall stones have been given a separate rubric.

THEMATIC REPERTORY
—By J.A. Mirrili - 1995

The author opines that it is very difficult to understand homoeopathy from the material available–clinical & pure materia medica and repertories. He has tried to express the thematic philosophy of the study of homoeopathic symptoms by organizing the symptoms of pure materia medica and repertory by themes. He says that repertories were the result of an attempt to classify the homeopathic symptoms so that they could be used in the clinic for quick reference, but they have several limitations.

i. The first limitation is that symptoms are severed and classified in alphabetical order with no connections in the repertory. Thus they loose their dynamic expression and similar symptoms are placed in different chapters remaining unrelated.

ii. Secondly, the symptoms described in pure materia medica are not totally represented in the reportorial rubrics.

Plan and Construction

In this new Thematic Repertory, author has tried to overcome the weaknesses of the repertories. For example, in the Thematic Repertory, under Forsaken, we have a lot of symptoms with the sense of Forsaken or implying Forsaken, but they do not resent the word Forsaken.

The Thematic Repertory incorporates the collected mood and 12,500 symptoms from the pure materia medicas of Hahnemann, Hering, T.F. Allen, H.C. Allen, Jeremy Sherr and the Complete Repertory by Roger Van Zandvoort.

These are arranged carefully under nearly 300 themes like Ambition, Forsaken, Death, Helplessness, Money, Religious, Travel, Yielding, etc. In this way, all the unrelated symptoms are present under the same theme and the limitation of the Kentian repertories, where similar symptoms with different spellings are found to be listed far away from each other is overcome.

ROBIN MURPHY'S REPERTORY OF HOMEOPATHIC MATERIA MEDICA

1. Plan and Construction

It was released in March 1993. It is a re-organized and expanded version of Kent's Repertory with the format of Kent and Knerr. The book is compact, practical and easy to carry like Kent's Repertory. It has 67 different chapters arranged alphabetically as compared to 37 in Kent's. Rubrics and sub-rubrics within each chapter are in an alphabetical format, similar to those of the materia medica leaving out Kent's plan of site, time, modalities, extensions, etc. There is complete reorganization of the information with smaller anatomical and functional subdivisions in alphabetical order. The grading of drugs is similar to Kent's three grades i.e., bold, bold italics and plain type.

2. Editions

The first edition of this repertory came in the year 1993. It has 67 chapters against 37 of Kent's. The basis of the first edition has been the whole of Kent's Repertory + large sections of Knerr's Repertory. The second edition appeared in 1996. Apart from a thorough revision of the first edition, it included 3 more chapters namely:

- Diseases
- Constitutions
- Headache

In addition to the 2 sources of the first edition already mentioned, the second edition includes symptoms from *Allen's Encyclopedia* and *Hering's Guiding Symptoms*. The third edition has come. The title has been changed to Homeopathic Clinical Repertory. It has 74 chapters.

3. Advantages over Kent's Repertory

Kent's Repertory is weak in information in respect to mental disorders, emergencies, infections, pathologies and when you have complaints relating to major organs. Murphy's repertory takes care of all these conditions. There are 40,000 new rubrics and 200 thousand new additions and updates, which include some of the new proving of Jeremy Sherr like Chocolate and Scorpion. In the end, there is a word index, which is very convenient for locating a particular rubric.

Following are some of the important chapters with the number of rubrics included under them mentioned against them:

Chapter   No. of rubrics included.

Diseases   450
Children   172
Emergencies   148
Environment   35
Pregnancy   140
Toxicity   72
Constitutions   76

Some of the important rubrics, which helps in selecting a remedy, are:

Goitre

Menses before aggravates – cimic.

Nodulated – *iod*.

Vertigo with – *iod.*

Goitre, exophthalmic

Grief from – aml-n.

Menses, after suppression of- **FERR**.

Tuberculosis, history with – dros.

Nerves, paralysis

Pseudo- hypotrophic – cur., phos., thyr., ver-v.

Weak muscles

Could hardly move about – ferr-p.

Raising arm to mouth is painful – eucal.
Sexual debility in – dig., ph-ac.

Pulse
Double pulse, angina pectoris in - aml-n.

Beats seem to run into each other – 1ber.
Feels pulse, in different parts of, in – nat-p.

Toxicity
Artificial foods, aggravates – alum., calc., mag-c., nat-p., sulph.
Chemotherapy, treatment, for side effects of – ars, CAD-S., chin., ip., nux-v.

Diseases
Myasthenia gravis – alum., con., gels.

Vitiligo - sep, thuj.

EXAMPLES OF CASES TREATED

Case—1

I may mention some cases wherein selection of a particular rubric helped in the prescription.

In the first case, the patient had a very marked symptom

"injustice, cannot tolerate". This rubric is only available in Murphy's Repertory and drugs mentioned are Causticum, Ignatia, Nux vomica, Plumbum and Staphysagria.

After differentiation among these drugs Nux vomica was selected which cured the case.

Case—2

An elderly patient had difficulty in swallowing the food as thick mucous prevented any swallowing. The rubric in Murphy's repertory "swallowing aggravate mucous from thick" suggested Alumina, Causticum and Sepia. On the basis of the other symptoms of the patient, Sepia was selected which gave prompt relief.

Case—3

A parent complained about his son who had a nasty habit of spitting on other peoples. It was embarrassing for the parents. A look in where Murphy's Repertory indicated a rubric " spit, desire to, faces of people in" where drugs like Arsenicum, **Belladonna**, Bufo, Cuprum, Stramonium and Veratrum were indicated. Presence of epileptic attacks led to the prescription of Bufo which considerably helped the patient.

Case—4

A patient of multiple sclerosis gave a definite history that his complaint started from grief. A rubric "multiple sclerosis, grief from", suggested the following drugs: Causticum, Conium, Phosphorus and Natrum mur. Natrum mur was chosen on the basis of some other symptoms of the case which helped the patient considerably.

Dr. Murphy has updated the language of the repertory in many places for which many new generations of homeopathic students will thank him many times. For example, "boredom" replaces "ennui", "crying" replaces "weeping" and "humiliation" replaces "mortification" though the original terms are cross referenced to the terms in updated language.

There is a bold reorganization and expansion of repertorial information with many practical divisions such as the ones having to do with children, pregnancy, emergencies, the environment, dreams and delusions including the use of modern diagnostic terminology as Alzheimer's syndrome, polycystic ovaries, etc.

He has created sections, which make it easier to locate an experience such as symptoms related to music, besides separate sections which have music as a modality. He has a music section in the Mind chapter, which includes many other mental symptoms, related to music.

There are plenty cross references and a very useful word index at the back of the book to locate difficult symptoms.

4. Drawbacks

It lacks the superscript code reference of the authors who have contributed towards addition to Kent. Therefore it is very difficult to know the source of the concerned data and remedy.

If we compare three rubrics of Murphy with that of Complete repertory in MacRepertory: "Deceitful", "Defiant" and "Ailments from reproaches". In "Deceitful" *Lycopodium (2), Opium (3)* and *Thuja (3)* are upgraded in Murphy's Repertory, in comparison to the Complete Repertory and *Morphinum* is added, with the other remedies in the rubric being identical. Again because of the absence of references, one does not know the source of these additions/upgrades.

In "Defiant", *Chamomilla (2)* and *Medorrhinum (1)* are added and *Tuberculinum* is upgraded (3), Again the same comments are applicable.

In "Ailments from reproaches", he has added *Anacardium*

(1), Chamomilla (1), Lycopodium (3) and *Natrium muriaticum (2)* and *upgraded Carcinosinum (2) Colocynthis (2)* and *Staphysagria (3).*

There are some rubrics which have been combined from the original Kent's Repertory. An example is combination of "egoistical" and "haughty" into one rubric entitled as "Egoistical haughty." The two words describe two distinct characteristics, as originally perceived by Kent, and belong to two separate rubrics.

COMPLETE REPERTORY BY ROGER VAN ZANDVOORT

1. Plan and Construction

This is the largest, most complete, and most accurate repertory in the history of homeopathy. It comes in three volumes: Mind, Vertigo through Speech and Voice and Respiration through Generalities and an all-in-one volume (2,830 pages). Using Kent's Repertory as the core, Van Zandvoort poured in the contents of every reliable repertory he could put his hands on, including the unique personal repertories of Pierre Schmidt and von Boenninghausen.

Zandvoort brought a millennium version of Complete Repertory, which is better than ever. It has 9000 new additions, 3000 new reference and cross-references, 33 new authors and 63 new remedies.

Zandvoort also created a multi-conceptual repertory known as *Repertory Universalis*. This is an integrated repertory which integrates the approaches of 3 masters of repertory namely Boenninghausen, Boger and Kent.

2. Sources of Complete Repertory

i. First, third, and sixth American editions of Kent's Repertory.

ii. Homeopathic journals.
iii. Schmidt's and Chand's Final General Repertory.
iv. Kunzli's Repertorium Generale.
v. Sivaraman's Additions and Corrections to Kent's Repertory.
vi. Boger's Additions to Kent's Repertory.
vii. Dr. Rastogi's Corrections to Abbreviations of Remedies used in Boenninghausen's Repertory [acknowledged as CCRH contribution].

Information and cross-references have been added from Pierre Schmidt's, Kent's, Boenninghausen's and Boericke's Repertories. The most useful part of Phatak's Repertory has been completely incorporated using reference works for cross-checking the material with their source.

There are about 515,000 confirmed additions in the Complete Repertory along with a number of new remedies: Ozone, Bambusa, Marble, Limestone, Sequoia sempervirens, Lac humanum, Hydrophis (snake venom), many additions from Saccharum officinalis, Carcinosinum and Bowel nosodes, Granite and Bothrops atrox. Each and every rubric has been traced to its origin mentioned in the superscript coded number giving the page number of the original text for each rubric for precision reference. This is the greatest advantage of this repertory as each new information has a reference code by which one can judge its value or worth.

There has been a lot of planning in the sectional organization of the repertory. The mind symptoms have been systematically classified and indexed so that the right rubric or remedy can be found easily. Noises in several sections have been brought together under the main rubric "Noise" (like in abdomen, grumbling, quacking, etc.).

He has changed previously confusing abbreviations to more

easily understood versions, mostly in the mineral and acid remedies.

Many symptoms have been simplified using the most common word for their specific meaning. The most important word in many rubrics has been moved at the beginning of the line, so that it can be read first; i.e. "during urination" is changed to "urination, during". The terminology in some cases has been modernized and clarified e.g. "miscarriage" has been replaced with "abortion" and "micturition" by "urination".

3. Some Important Changes

One example of a rubric in Mind section: Emotions predominated by intellect (as it appears in Synthetic Repertory) has been changed to, after confirmation from text to: Emotions-Controlled by intellect, need to be. This phrasing of the rubric gives it exactly the opposite meaning. Whereas the first one indicates that the intellect is so strong that it overwhelms and controls the emotions, the actual meaning indicates that emotions are so strong that they have to be controlled by intellect. The latter makes sense because the drugs enlisted against the rubric (Valer. and Viol-o.) are known to be highly emotional and hysterical drugs and not intellectual ones as depicted earlier.

The latest edition of Complete Repertory also adds another rubric:

Emotions, too strong – which also has the same drugs. This again confirms the corrections.

Some of the new rubrics are: Ability increased, Achieve things desire to, Animal consciousness, Borrows trouble, Blaming, Charitable, Constructive, Daydreaming, Delicacy feeling of, Dignity, Housekeeping inept for, Independent, Enthusiasm, Teasing, Telepathy, Intellectual.

A number of sub-rubrics have been added:

Precocity – religious, sexual, school, but does not perform to capacity.

Embraces – trees wants to embrace: ozone.

Extravagance – economy for want of, sometimes miserly, works hard.

Consolation refuses for one's own: Nitric acid.

Contemptuous – opponent for, relations for, society.

4. Disadvantages

i. A lot of unreliable additions have been made, both in terms of drugs and rubrics; e.g., Androctonus and Chocolate are two drugs which are put in almost all rubrics.

ii. Lot of cross references, which turn out to be futile.

iii. Many small rubrics with single drugs lead the prescriber to go astray if given too much importance.

iv. It weighs almost 10 kg, making it difficult to carry.

SYNTHESIS: REPERTORIUM HOMEOPATHICUM SYNTHETICUM
—By Frederik Schroyens

Synthesis is the Repertory linked to the RADAR project. It is based on the sixth American edition of Kent's Repertory and contains all its rubrics and remedies. Since 1987, Synthesis has been used as a database for the RADAR program in the daily practice of leading homeopaths. It has been commented upon and thereby improved over and over again, which gives it an outstanding label of quality. This repertory is the best example of the expanded version of Kent's Repertory from 1916 till date. It retains the Kent's hierarchical structure, therefore there is no need to learn a new format. It incorporates a vast number of corrections and adaptations caused by textual errors, illogical symptoms, locations and ambiguous wordings found in original e.g., breast is replaced by mammae or chest when appropriate. There are about 235,000 additions from highly respected homeopathic texts, giving priority to the classical authors – Kent, Hahnemann, Hering, Allen, Clarke, Boericke, Knerr, etc.

- The sole aim remains to enhance transparency, consistency and readability.
- Its goal has been quality of information.
- Synthesis contains repeated checked additions from the homeopathic literature including Hahnemann, Kent, Hering, Allen, Clarke, Boericke, Knerr, etc.
- Additions from living authors are added only with caution and most often, only in the first degree unless confirmation (of a higher degree) comes from other authors.
- Thousands of corrections to Kent's Repertory have been made. They are recognizable as the remedy in these cases mentions "K" as well as the reference.
- Thousands of symptoms have been rewritten following a clearly readable "symptom format" e.g., "pieces, sensation as if head would fall in, when stooping became " pieces, in stooping", sensation as if head would fall in".
- Wherever possible ambiguous words have been clarified.
- Spellings have been changed like "anaemia" became "anemia", "diarrhoea" became "diarrhea".
- Clinical rubrics were renamed according to modern disease names e.g., "coryza –annual" became "hayfever", skin- becomes sore" became "decubitus".
- A new list of author abbreviations and a new standard list of remedy abbreviations has been given.
- It appeared in 1993.
- Version 4 contains 178,000 additions to Kent.
- Version 5 had 181,000 more additions.

- Version 7 contains 235,000 more additions collected from more than 330 different sources.
- There is a catalogue of 3712 remedies in Version 7, while in Version 8.1 the number of remedies has become 4200.
- Version 8.1 contains 2277 remedies.
- Version 9.1 contains 2373 remedies.

Synthesis 9.1 version is the latest [2088 pages] and incorporates the repertories of Boger, Boenninghausen, Boericke and Phatak. The theme of Synthesis 9.1 seems to be streamlining and restructuring and there are 3 extra chapters: Neck, Urinary Organs and Female/Male Genitalia.

GENTRY'S REPERTORY

This is a repertory aimed at finding a particular symptom of our materia medica.

The symptoms are arranged in such a way that they can be located by using a noun, adjective or verb of the symptom.

It can be described as a word search repertory.

It was published in 1890, the second edition came 1892.

1. Origin of This Repertory

i. **Once in 1876, Dr. Gentry had a case which presented a unique under mentioned symptom:**

" Constant dull frontal headache, worse in the temples with aching in the umbilicus."

Dr. Gentry spent several hours to locate this symptom in the materia medica as he did not find in the repertories. This gave him the idea of creating a repertory where this symptom could be searched easily by looking under "U" that is to say, umbilicus.

He included more characteristic pathogenetic symptoms and only repeatedly verified symptoms.

ii. This repertory is made, to enable the physician to find quickly and certainly, the desired symptom in the materia medica together with the indicated remedy.

2. Rules Adopted for Construction

i. Select and give all the nouns, verbs and essential adjectives in the sentence.

ii. Where two or more remedies have the power of producing a similar condition, include them as merely suggestive.

3. Usefulness

i. The utility of this repertory is limited to word search.
ii. It is not created to repertorize the case.
iii. The job of word search is now-a-days best done by computerized softwares of various repertories.
iv. One symptom can be referred at many places, E.g. confusion in head, which makes thinking difficult can be found under Head and also under Mind.
v. It has 420 remedies.

4. Volumes

There are 6 volumes.

Volume I contains:

- Mind and Disposition
- Head
- Eyes
- Ears

- Nose
- Face

Volume II contains:
- Mouth
- Throat
- Stomach
- Hypochondria

Volume III contains:
- Abdomen
- Anus
- Rectum and Stool
- Urine and urinary Organs
- Male Sexual System

Volume IV contains:
- Uterus and Appendages
- Menstruation and Discharges
- Pregnancy and Parturition
- Lactation and Mammary Glands

Volume V contains:
- Voice, Larynx and Trachea
- Chest, Lungs, Bronchi and Cough
- Heart and Circulation
- Chill and Fever
- Skin, Sleep and Dreams

Volume VI contains:
- Neck and Back

- Upper Extremities
- Lower Extremities
- Bones and Limbs in General
- Nerves
- Generalities and Keynotes

5. Important Features

i. All the characteristic and pathognomic symptoms are given.
ii. It includes only repeatedly verified clinical symptoms.
iii. Phraseology of the materia medica has been used, E.g. under catamania there are few drugs whereas, under menses there are many.

Some Examples

- Desire to kiss everybody

We can view this under the followings:

Mind and Disposition: Wants

Mind and Disposition : Kiss

Mind and Disposition: Everybody

Mind and Disposition: Desire

- Constant, dull aching in umbilical region, with frontal headache at same time

We can view this under:

The abdomen: Aching

The abdomen: Headache

The abdomen: Umbilical region

Head and scalp: Frontal

INTEGRATED HOMOEOPATHIC REPERTORY OF MIND
—By Dr. Jugal Kishore

The integrated repertory [Mind] is from one of the most brilliant homeopathic physicians having profound knowledge of the subject besides having a vast clinical experience. He is known for his consistent views. Thus I have known his views on integrating anatomy and physiology at the undergraduate level and integrating relevant topics of modern medicine at the postgraduate level. I have also known him to judge things from a practical angle. Therefore, there is no surprise that he has produced this repertory by integrating Boenninghausen's approach with that of Kent's, applying the concept of analogy to mental symptoms. The result is a brilliant repertory, rich in verified rubrics, which will surely help in locating the curative remedy. There is no doubt that there was a need of a reliable repertory of this kind.

Dr. Kishore has taken us to the roots or back to the basic repertory which is the mother of all repertories and added more rubrics and remedies from Synthetic, Knerr, Boger, Boenninghausen, J.H. Clarke, Phatak, Boericke and Vithoulkas, apart from his own vast and rich clinical experience.

Dr. Kishore has added 'Time, Aggravations and Ameliorations' on the pattern of BBR.

However on checking, I found some differences in the placement of remedies. For example, take the rubric "Cloudy weather aggravates". In BBR, the remedies Am-c. and Phos. are shown in italics while in the Integrated Repertory, these are shown in ordinary type.

I looked up another rubric 'constipation' aggravates. In BBR, it is listed as 'constipation during', while in Integrated Homoeopathic Repertory of Mind, it is changed to 'constipation when' and there is a change in placement of remedies as Nux-v. has not been shown in italics while Calc. and Psor. are added in italics.

The strength of this repertory is the immense credibility of the author and his rich experience.

INTEGRATED HOMOEOPATHIC REPERTORY OF GENERALITIES

—By Dr. Jugal Kishore

This provides a revolutionary approach to the study of repertory and includes an exhaustive and unusual collection of physical generals with modalities affecting man as a whole.

It covers 686 pages of generalities as compared to 387 pages of Synthetic and 82 pages of Kent. Boericke's Materia Medica and Repertory are included besides multiple other repertories and materia medicas.

MINI REPERTORIES

Mini repertories on the following are available:
1. Cancerous affections.
2. Tuberculosis.
3. Prophylactics.
4. Tissues: Bones, Joints, Muscles, Mucous membranes and Nerves.

Remedies of the sub-rubrics are added to the main rubrics to avoid missing the indicated remedy.

SOME CLINICAL REPERTORIES

CLINICAL REPERTORY
—By Oscar Eugene Boericke

This repertory was first published in 1906, along with the third edition of William Boericke's Materia Medica.

Later in 1927, it was completely remodeled and brought up to date in its ninth edition.

It includes 1407 drugs.

1. *Gradations*

There are two grades:

        Italics   : 2 marks
        Romans : 1 mark

2. Arrangement of Chapters in the Repertory

i. Under each chapter the rubrics are arranged in an alphabetical order.

ii. Rubrics in each chapter are printed in bold capitals.

iii. Sub-rubrics are printed in roman bold at first indentation. Sub rubrics are also arranged alphabetically.

iv. Cross-references are given after remedies for the particular rubric or sub-rubric.

v. After rubrics and sub-rubrics, clinical condition or synonyms are given in parenthesis.

vi. Arrangement of sub-rubrics is as follows:

- Cause.
- Type.
- Location.
- Character.
- Concomitants.
- Modalities.

The repertory has 24 chapters:

I.	Mind	XIII.	Stomach
II.	Head	XIV.	Abdomen
III.	Eyes	XV.	Urinary system
IV.	Ears	XVI.	Male sexual system
V.	Nose	XVII.	Female sexual system
VI.	Face	XVIII.	Locomotor system
VII.	Mouth	XIX.	Respiratory system
VIII.	Tongue	XX.	Skin
IX.	Taste	XXI.	Fever
X.	Gums	XXII.	Nervous system
XI.	Teeth	XXIII.	Generalities
XII.	Throat	XXIV.	Modalities: Aggravations and Ameliorations

A CLINICAL REPERTORY TO THE DICTIONARY OF MATERIA MEDICA

—By John Henry Clarke

The first Edition was published in 1904.

It is constructed on the basis of "Dictionary of Practical Materia Medica".

1. Plan and Construction

i. This repertory consists of five parts:
- Clinical Repertory.
- Repertory of Causation.
- Repertory of Constitution, Temperament, Disposition and States.
- Repertory of Clinical Relationship.
- Repertory of Natural Relationship.

ii. In this repertory, the author has followed Cypher Repertory for remedy abbreviations.

e.g., for acids "X" is used, like "Nt. X", "Fl. X", etc.

iii. The repertory includes 1067 drugs which are arranged in two gradations.

iv. The rubrics are arranged in an alphabetical order in all the five parts.

v. Every time a medicine is mentioned, it begins with a capital letter. When a name has two parts the second part always starts with a small letter.

THE HOMOEOPATHIC THERAPEUTICS OF DIARRHAE
—By James B.Bell

The book has basically two parts:

Part I : Remedies and their indications. Number of drugs included are 141

Part II : Repertory.

1. Gradation of Drugs

BOLD — 1st grade
Italics — 2nd grade
Roman — 3rd grade
(Roman) — 4th grade

2. The format of Repertory

The Repertory has been divided into five parts:
i. Pathological Names
ii. Character of Stools
iii. Condition of stool and accompanying symptoms
   - Aggravation
   - Amelioration
iv. Accompaniments of evacuation
   - Before stool
   - During stool
   - After stool
v. General accompaniments: This part has 23 sub-sections. They are arranged according to the Hahnemannian schema.

COMPLETE REPERTORY TO THE HOMOEOPATHIC MATERIA MEDICA
—By E.W. Berridge

The book deals with the "Diseases of the Eyes" only.

Actually this repertory first appeared in the homoeopathic Journal "The Hahnemannian Monthly". It should be considered as the first edition. In 1873, the second edition was published where its volume was enormously enlarged. Its size became almost double that of the first edition.

1. Format of the Repertory

The repertory is arranged as follows:

Section I: Symptoms
i. Functions
ii. Anatomical Regions
iii. General Character, Sequence, Direction

    iv. Right Side (Right Eye)
    v. Left Side (Left Eye)

Section II : Conditions
    i. Aggravations
    ii. Ameliorations

THE THERAPEUTICS OF INTERMITTENT FEVER
—By Henry C. Allen

The book consists of four parts:
1. Introduction
2. Therapeutic Part
3. Repertory Proper
4. Abbreviations and Remedies

The Repertory Part
    i. Type
    ii. Time
    iii. Cause
    iv. Prodrome
    v. Commencement of chill
    vi. Heat
    vii. Sweat
    viii. Tongue, appetite, taste, etc.
    ix. Apyrexia, symptoms during

PATHOGENETIC AND CLINICAL REPERTORY OF HEAD
—By Charles Neidhard

This repertory was compiled from *Allen's Encyclopedia of Materia Medica*. To this the clinical verifications and experiences of the author's fifty years of homeopathic practice have been added.

COMPUTERIZED REPERTORIES

RADAR
(Rapid Aid to Drug Aimed Research)

It is one of the best softwares for windows. It uses Synthesis 7 which incorporates all the work of the Synthesis team world wide since June 1993. All the new proving from Jeremy Sherr's Dynamis Volume I, plus many other new proving have been added in it. There is accurate information on over 2000 remedies; there are 260,000 additions from 320 different sources as compared to Kent (approximately 1844 pages). Analysis can be personalized as there are several ways of analyzing the rubrics which also include the Vithoulkas Expert System.

Radar 8 has introduced the function of Confidence Levels. Every homeopath can decide for himself which Minimum Confidence Level is to be used, the higher the Minimum Confidence Level, the less information is displayed, but the more trustworthy this information will be. With version 8.2 one now gets full control over a number of parameters. If one wishes, one can set them on their own.

Radar 8.2 also comes with new repertories which can be obtained and used separately from the Synthesis. The first one which is available is the *"Therapeutic Pocket Book"* by Boenninghausen (b2), in English and in German.

With the development of a new comprehensive Remedy-Families Database, it is easier than ever to investigate remedy concordances.

A more flexible implementation of the Synthesis Additions Password has been programmed, avoiding the situation where people would get blocked when making many additions.

Radar 9.2 has the distinct advantage of using Boger, Boenninghausen, Boericke, Phatak, Boger's Synoptic Key, Boger's General Analysis, H.A. Roberts Sensation As If and Wards Sensation As If repertories exclusively. Besides it provides the facility of viewing additions made to Kent's Repertory by Vithoulkas, Sivaraman and Kunzli.

One can easily find out what has been recently added to the Archibel website by checking the *"What's New"* section.

1. Synthesis 9

What's New in Synthesis 9?

i. **Synthesis 9 (May 2004) is another milestone in the development of homeopathic repertories.**
   - Synthesis 9 contains more than 300,000 additions as opposed to the previous Version 8.
   - Synthesis 9 is a voluminous homeopathic repertory (more than 1 million rubrics).

ii. **Substantial new information.**
   - From Andre Saine (Canada) more than 3,200 clinical rubrics taken.
   - From Boericke, Materia Medica symptoms from the description of the characteristics and the Mind section. More than 14,700 additions.
   - From Julian's Materia Medica of the Nosodes.
   - From Master Farokh's Clinical Observation of Children's Remedies. More than 10,600 additions have been made from it.

iii. **Addition of three new chapters in Synthesis 9.1**
- Outer neck & throat (a chapter that Boenninghausen used in the Systematic Alphabetical Repertory).
- Urinary organs (symptoms like modalities, that refer to the urinary organs as a whole / totality).
- Genitalia & Sexuality (symptoms that can be applied to both the sexes in the same measure. Boger out of the same reason hasn't specified any sex organ).

Important: This web update is available for free for all latest version users.

2. *Concepts and Themes*

Translate the language of your patient into the language of the repertory. Patient may not provide the most accurate words to describe how he or she is feeling. It is up to the practitioner to recognize patterns, symptoms or key words during the interview process. This can sometimes make diagnosis very difficult for a homeopath, due to the fact that we are all very different, and our language leaves room for much uncertainty around the 'concept' of the patient's problem.

RADAR's "Concepts" is a unique tool that helps to translate the language of your patients into the language of the repertory. "Concepts" spider-like web of information connects rubrics based on themes or concepts. Now you can find the rubric that truly matches your patients' condition or be directed towards rubrics you never knew existed. With Concepts, finding any symptom in the repertory is as easy as a few simple mouse clicks.

Concepts' spider-like web of information stretches through the entire Synthesis Repertory, part of the RADAR program, considerably simplifying the search for symptoms by using the words and expressions of the patient as a point of departure. A click of the mouse is sufficient to display all the symptoms related to a

There are numerous books available for Concepts. Each book groups symptoms by different ideas or themes. Now you can find every rubric of chronic and acute disease conditions, which in the past may have taken many hours, or even days to locate. Concepts represents a revolutionary advancement by increase ease and use of homeopathic repertories.

3. *Encyclopedia Homeopathica*

EH 2.1 and later versions offer new search possibilities and an empty document for use. The world's largest, most reliable and structured Multilingual Homeopathic Reference Library - currently in 7 languages It includes more than 200,000 pages of homeopathic literature

More than 681 titles – A comprehensive library of classic and modern literature, including the work of George Vithoulkas, Jan Scholten, Alphonse Geukens, Franz Vermeulen, Frederik Schroyens, Roger Morrison, Nancy Herrick, Rajan Sankaran, Bill Gray, Jonathan Shore, Robin Murphy, Ananda Zaren and Lou Klein.

EH has amazed the homeopathic community with its accurate search results. Indeed, it is useful to have a lot of documents, but the search function defines which information you will find. With this new version, the powerful search engine has been further improved.

Now we find all articles written by the author of our choice. We will be able to find remedies based on their themes for the first time, with this version and with package H4 (English).

We will be able to import our own text into an empty document. If we follow some basic formatting rules, we can define a chapter; define to which remedy the text belongs, etc. Afterwards EH will find our text as well as the original documents when we search (for example) for that remedy.

Also the navigation has further improved. Shortcuts have been added to help move quickly from one piece of information to another. In the Family Analysis Window, plus and minus signs in front of the families clearly indicate where a family can be expanded or collapsed. In the Symptom Clipboard, the words of the hits are now highlighted.

i. Scientific Searches

The database of Encyclopedia Homeopathica is unique in its quality and precision. Encyclopedia Homeopathica is the only program that has included all information from the texts in a coded format. For example, all prover indications in Allen's Encyclopedia or Hahnemann's Materia Medica are included. This allows the practitioner or student to check the exact origin of symptoms, which is essential for proper understanding of the original proving information. For example, in several remedies in Allen's Encyclopedia, the symptoms listed are a mixture of several sub-species. This information is of vital importance to be able to make reliable prescriptions or additions to the repertory.

ii. Great Flexibility

Encyclopedia Homeopathica provides the ability to quickly find the position of any remedy within the analysis. All search queries and analysis results can be exported to other programs or printed. Encyclopedia Homeopathica contains the entire contents of each book and journal, including proving information, footnotes and references. By presenting the remedy information in its original context with all comments and relevant information, the students and practitioners can glean a deeper understanding from these homeopathic jewels.

4. Kenbo

i. This software is designed to take every symptom of all the histories (present, past, personal, examination) of the patient.
ii. Automatic conversion of symptoms to rubrics found in various repertories (kent, boenninghausen, boger and boericke).
iii. Encouraging thorough case recording. All symptoms of the

patient are recorded in separate history screens and converted into rubrics.

iv. Display of rubrics for various clinical conditions which are not found in repertories, (like diabetes, renal failure, hypertension, ischemic heart disease, etc.)

v. Case analysis and evaluation of symptoms as per concept of drs. Hahnemann and kent.

vi. Ascertaining miasm for each symptom and deciding the dominant and fundamental miasm of the case.

vii. Display of sequential totality of case and creating conceptual image of case.

viii. Exclusive case proforma which automatically guides users for recording every important symptom of the case.

ix. Recording of subjective and objective symptoms, constitution and appearance, gestures of patients and converting them in to rubrics.

x. Suggestion of repertory on the basis of type of case.

xi. Formation of repertorial syndrome on the basis of quality of symptoms.

xii. Very fast repertorization of the case along with suggestions for & single simillimum, dose, potency and repetetion.

xiii. Selection of simillimum on the basis of repertorial totality, underlying miasm and potential drug field.

xiv. Suggestions for intercurrent remedies.

xv. Future follow up of case according to kent's 12 observations and hering's law of cure.

xvi. Display of remedy relationship in follow up.

xvii. Mantain all account information, billing, besides generating various certificates.

xviii. Very useful for research purpose as it mantains seperate records of case groups.

xix. Mantains an appointment diary.
xx. Online study of materia medica.
xxi. Quick repertorisation and fastest search for any rubric in repertories.
xxii. User can also use simple repertorization as done in all other softwares.

If one desires to work with only 4 basic repertories namely Kent, Boericke, Boger and Boenninghausen, this is a useful program.

REFERENCE WORKS

Professional Version 2.0 and later

Published by David Kent Warkentin and Kent Homeopathic Associates, November 1995.

It is available for Mac as well as IBM, is a computer program.

It is a library of all the main materia medica (including medicine specific information from modern writers such as Sankaran, Scholten, Zaren, etc.) plus materia medica formed from all the main repertories and materia medica, some that come from journals that have not seen the light of day for many a years. It is more than this as it can be directly used to analyse cases. This is a unique facility and extremely useful in practice.

Different Ways to use Reference Works

i. **Like a library**
One can go to any section of any medicine in any materia medica or repertory generated materia medica. It contains all information except introduction and general comment about the drugs. There is an easy and useful bookmark system that means you keep track and go back to any text by placing a marker on the page in the materia medica window. It also includes Zizia philosophy containing Hahnemann's Organon, Kent's Philosophy, Robert's

Principles and Stuart Close's Genius of Homoeopathy.

ii. **Find rare symptoms in difficult cases**

One can scan the entire literature for occurrence of any rare symptom in the text, which is usually not listed in any repertory. For example I wanted to see the oldest reference of the term "cervical spondylosis" in homeopathic source books. I gave this command in Reference work and found that the term has been specifically used under the drug Phosphoricum acidum by Hering, and is also mentioned in Knerr's Repertory.

iii. **Find more complete rubrics**

Almost in all common routinely used rubrics like desire and aversion, one finds a number of additions as compared to the limited ones in a routine repertories.

One can see the relevant words in sentence or paragraph or a remedy.

iv. **Selective search for words and books**

v. **Analyze cases**

Use the materia medica as a huge repertory.

vi. **Make your own materia medica of clinical uses**

vii. **Exporting information of Mac Repertory**

CARA & SIMILIA

Two new softwares with the name of CARA & SIMILIA have been developed in England. Miccant, UK now ISIS-Inspirational software.

1. CARA

CARA is a repertory software, which has certain new features of browsing between repertories and making a combined search between repertories. It tells us about properties of drugs besides having an expert system for analysis. It also helps users to add new rubrics and one can create one's own repertory.

CARA provides Kent's Repertory, Synthetic Repertory, Boericke's Repertory, Phatak's Materia Medica, Kent's Lectures and Allen's Keynotes all as standard. It also includes in the repertory all the additions to Kent suggested by Vithoulkas, provings of Scorpion, Hydrogen, Adamas, Brassica, Germanium, Eagle, Iridium, Neon and Chocolate made by Dynamis school. The recognized additions for Carcinosinum are also included. It also includes a variety of materia medica and the Complete Repertory.

2. SIMILIA

SIMILIA is a computer program that brings materia medica and philosophy textbooks on to our computer screen, providing instant access to the writings of both classical and contemporary homeopathic physicians. For details of books see Annexure C.

HOMPATH

This software was developed in India by Dr. Jawahar Shah and is being improved in speed and features. It is also being converted from DOS to Window version. Its several special features are available as a whole as well as in parts. Hompath Classic Version 7.0 runs on Mac and PC's, and incorporates more than 250 books including the Complete Repertory by Roger Van Zandvoort. Hompath Ozone runs only on PC's and contains three books including Kent's and Boericke's Repertory. Hompath Win is for PC's and Hompath ST is also for PC's (Dos version). Both contain 24 repertories, 4 materia medicas along with 10,000 cross-references. Materia Medica Live runs on PC's and Mac; has a Multimedia presentation CD, for 22 remedies. Now, Version 8 has come which has superceded all its precursors in user friendliness and utility.

Classic version 8.0 is chiefly a product for the practicing classical homeopath. It contains more than 300 books covering a wide range of homeopathic subjects. It has easy graphic interface, and is intuitive to learn. It includes numerous unique and new features.

Features

i. 300 books : Book list (Authors arranged in alphabetical order).

ii. Quick repertorization:
   An instant repertorization module is present which allows you to repertorize while the patient narrates has/her symptoms. All repertorization options and filters available on same screen.

iii. Group symptoms:
   - Analyse symptoms based on groups.
   - Learn more about remedies by creating 'group symptoms' of specific groups.
   - Make statistical remedy and symptom analysis a feature significant to researchers.

iv. Confirmation of symptoms:
   Confirm symptoms and remedies of repertories from materia medica source books.

v. Quick search:
   Fast and exact search / recording of symptoms, accessing specific chapters and rubrics directly.

vi. Combined symptoms repertory:
   Combine two or more symptoms to record it for repertorisation or save it as a combined symptom repertory.

vii. Advanced search options:
   - Normal, essential and vital words to improve your search criteria thereby ensuring accurate and complete results.

- Search query of repertory words – Search repertory words from materia medica and Tresorie, from one screen itself.
- Language options – American and British English, singular and plural words, are taken care of in search results thereby not missing out because of different language words.

viii. Intelligent search:
- Cross-references.
- Themes.
- Similar words.
- Synonyms.
- Word meanings.

ix. Search / record from all these options. Rubric hunting and recording made simple and easy:

x. Improves your knowledge of rubrics, helps you to consider symptoms, which you would have otherwise missed:

xi. Materia medica repertory:

A unique and novel feature, which allows you to create a repertory from the materia medica and thereafter repertorize using this repertory.

xii. Symptoms forwarding:

Forward symptoms from previous cases to new and current cases

thereby saving time on re-repertorisation.

xiii. Rubrics related:
- Great interlinking of cross-references, themes, synonyms, word meanings and similar words for rubrics.
- Accessible from all the modules wherever the symptoms or rubrics are present.

xiv. Remedy related:

- Great interlinking of drug property, drug relations, Keynotes and materia medica for the drugs.
- Accessible from all the modules wherever the remedies are available.

xv. Interlinked feature:

All modules are interlinked beautifully making it possible to jump from one module to another without having to close any module.

Classic has a comprehensive Repertory and Materia Medica Search which is intelligent, fast and useful. It provides insight into a never before knowledge of remedy portraits and rubric occurrences. There are smart, intelligent and practical repertorization strategies and expert analysis based on rules laid down by Masters of homeopathy - Kent, Boenninghausen and Boger. Remedy analysis by various filters—animal, mineral and plant kingdoms. An added feature is that it offers 5000 pages of Gentry's Concordances, Phatak's Repertory and many more other repertories, which make finding the true simillimum very easy. This software comes with a built-in *Patient Analysis*, which enables physicians to improve patient management.

A new version has been brought under the name Hompath Vital. It contains 21000 pages of information from 100 books and has 5 repertories namely Kent, Boericke, Boger, Boenninghausen and Phatak, and includes features of Classic 8.0. Another version has come known as HOMPATH MD.

HOMEOPATHIC REPERTORIZATION SYSTEM (HRS)

Homeopathic Repertorization System is a simple program of Kent's Repertory, Allen's Keynotes and Hering's Guiding Symptoms. You simply have to choose the symptoms from various repertory chapters, and a graph will come up. In Allen's Keynotes, it has the facility to browse between different remedies coming into relationships on the same screen.

PHOENIX REPERTORY

The Phoenix Repertory is based on Kent's Repertory Format, having 38 chapters (37 chapters as per Kent Repertory and one new chapter on dreams). Dreams chapter is separated from sleep as dream represent our emotions, so this chapter has been placed after Mind chapter.

Rubrics are placed alphabetically in each chapter in the order of Side, Time, Modality, Extension and Localization.

Features

i. The 80,000 additions have been made from 540 different sources, from Hahnemann to Rajan Sankaran.

ii. Most of these corrections were collected from Reference works and many have never been included before in any repertory.

iii. More than 20,000 corrections have been made from Kent's Repertory (Dr. Diwan Harishchand and Dr. R.P. Patel). Corrections have been suggested by Sivaraman (CCRH corrections to Boenninghausen repertory).

iv. New rubrics have been added. There is a need to add more rubrics because many a times you don't find appropriate expression of the symptom you are looking for in your case. So, new rubric phrases were created from other repertories and materia medicas.

v. New remedies. In recent years, much work has been done by different homeopathic teachers and organizations in new provings, re-provings and clinical verification of remedies. Valuable suggestions have been incorporated in the Phoenix

Repertory.
vi. Different personalities with proper cross-references.
vii. Phobia terms are cross-referenced with rubrics of fear.
viii. Medical conditions are added.
ix. New synonymous cross-references are created.

All remedy additions and rubrics include original author ID. When you need to know exactly how a remedy manifests a certain symptom using exact author abbreviations, you can go to the exact book and author.

PHATAK'S REPERTORY

It is one of the most reliable alphabetical repertory. Dr. Phatak has included rubrics duly verified by him. This repertory does not take the place of exhaustive repertories like Kent's or Boenninghausen's but is very concise and practical. For its construction, Dr. Phatak relied on the following authorities:

Dr. Boger
Dr. Kent
Dr. Clarke

This is no doubt a handy and useful reference book to lessen the difficulties of the prescriber.

KENTIAN HOMEOPATHIC COMPUTER PROGRAM

It is a program designed on the corrected version of Kent's Repertory by Dr. R.P. Patel.

It has the following advantages:

i. There are three ways to enter patient's symptoms to repertorize for quick and easy time saving procedures :
  - Directly through chapters of Kent's Repertory.
  - Directly through code numbers of the rubrics.

- Search facility: Its advance search engine helps one to find out the exact rubric(s) from the entire Kent's Repertory by typing the word or the rubric.

ii. It automatically does the following after entering patient's selected symptoms for repertorization :
    - Classify patient's symptom(s) according to Kent's analysis of symptoms in order of hierarchy even if symptoms are entered haphazardly.
    - Evaluates patient's symptoms according to Hahnemann, Kent and others.
    - Classify the more striking, singular, uncommon and peculiar (characteristic) signs and symptoms according to § 153 of the Organon.
    - Classify symptoms of the three miasms according to Hahnemann.
    - Classify all important symptoms through the built in homeopathic expert system to arrive at the correct remedy.

iii. There are several innovative ways to repertorise.
    - Normal or flat type of repertorization.
    - RUPS –Rare, uncommon, peculiar, strange or artistic way of repertorization.
    - Miasmatic basis of repertorization.
    - Homeopthic expert system method.

This is a very simple and straight forward program to work with if one wants to limit repertorization to Kent's Repertory.

ISIS V2

This is known as the Inspirational Software, also developed by David Witko and was released in 2003. Its ease of use and sophisticated features made it a favorite soon.

This is a software which combines repertory, materia medica, remedies data base and dictionary in one. Its easy to use interface and this is the most appealing advantage of this software.

It is not an upgrade of CARA as is commonly believed. It is a completely new program, which has been designed by David Witko for the homeopathic practitioner and is pretty easy to use. It includes practically everything that is needed like searching rubrics, materia medica information, various strategies of repertorizing like through families, miasms, and the concept of Sankaran, etc. The display of charts is beautiful. Even simple browsing of the repertory or remedy database is most fascinating. The dictionary provides meanings of words relevant to homeopathic concepts / context, which is very useful in understanding. Finding or locating a rubric is most easy.

ISIS contains the following repertories:

i. The classic repertories: Boericke, Phatak, Boenninghausen and Clarke.

ii. Contemporary repertories It also contains the contemporary repertories namely Combined Repertory by Miccant LTD, Complete Repertory by Roger Van Zandvoort and Homeopathic Medical Repertory by Robin Murphy. The Repertorium Universalis by Zandvoort can be added.

A new version has come which is known as ISIS VISION from Miccant's ISIS system. This version adds speed, power and flexibility.

CORRECTIONS OF ABBREVIATIONS FOR MEDICINES USED IN BOGER-BOENNINGHAUSEN'S REPERTORY

D. P. Rastogi and V. D. Sharma

SUMMARY

This paper presents the results of correcting the abbreviations used in the Boger Boenninghausen's Repertory, to bring them in line with the abbreviation which are used in Kent's work. In the process of checking, several (about 100) errors in the name of the drugs were noted. The correct names of of drugs were identified after a thorough search in authoritative works.

This paper presents the errors and suggested corrections and reference. It is hoped that with the incorporation of these corrections the value of this monumental work would be further increased.

Key word: Repertory, Boenninghausen Boger, Abbreviation errors.

Although, Hahnemann was the first person who felt the need of a repertory, the credit for creating the first repertory goes to Boenninghausen. *The Repertory of the Antipsoric Remedies* was created by Boenninghausen in 1832 and this was the repertory that Hahnemann used in his practice. Boenninghausen worked on making a small concise pocket book of his major work and, in 1846, came out with the *Therapeutic Pocket-Book*. This became the standard reference work used by most American homeopaths including Stuart Close, Carroll Dunham, H.N. Guernsey and T.F. Allen.

In 1900 Cyrus Boger made a new translation of the Repertory of the Antipsoric Remedies into English. It contained 232 pages. He continued to enhance it until his death in 1935. He made so many additions and new rubrics that its final size was 1040 pages; an almost fivefold increase. It is probably more correct to call this Boger's although it is known as Boger-Boenninghausen's Characteristics and Repertory (BBR).

This masterpiece however fell into comparative disuse because it had long lists of drugs in various rubrics and thus required a pretty long time to write down the drugs during repertorization. Thanks to the efforts of David Warkentin and his team, this useful work in available to users of the Mac Repertory programme. It has been my belief that if computerization is deemed necessary for the use of any repertory, the Boger-Boenninghausen Repertory needs it the most.

In the process of going through the various abbreviations of drugs used under various rubrics for undertaking computerization of this repertory we came across the following abbreviations of drugs under various caterogires of rubrics which could be put under the following groups:

- Abbreviations that did not point to any drug, for example: ars, euh, rhzn-c, mgs. s, berg, cimb, merg, crp, medx, aur-p, mex, carb-b, saes, tap, agaf, calac, saro, turb, sen-ac, pyso, cut-h, senio, pip-in phs, stup, pyng, caun, carb-m, etc.

- Abbreviations that were unclear and pointed to more than one drug. For example sol, manganese, amy stro, arum, mer, mag, can, org, chimp, cimb, can, crocc-c, ver-b, chena etc.

- Some of the abbreviations which could not be understood as no reference could be found in recorded books of provings. For example : Cioc, eucl, hychat, rups, id, etc.

The above abbreviations were carefully read and re-read and the probable drugs were screened through the various standard works like Hering's Guiding Symptoms, A Handbook of Materia Medica, Clarke's Materia Medica, Boger's Synoptic Key, Boericke's Materia Medica, Kent's Repertory (Kunzlï), Clinical Materia Medica by E.A. Farrington, and H.C. Allen's Nosodes and Keynotes. When a particular reference had been found for the probable drug it was also seen whether it corresponded to the alphabetical frame of the various other drugs given under the given rubric. Details of this exercise are presented in the following pages. For the corrections the Indian Edition of the BBR was used.

Abbreviations:

A.E.	Allen's Encyclopedia
Boe.	Boericke's Materia Medica
C.M.M.	Clarke's Materia Medica
H.G.S.	Hering's Guiding Symptoms.
Ch. Dis.	Hahnemann's Chronic Diseases
Boenning	Boenninghausen's Repertory
M.M. Pura	Hahnemann's Materia Medica Pura

Sl. no.	Abbr. of drugs given in Boger Boenninghausen's Repertory & Page No.	Rubric in Boger Boenninghausen's Repertory & Page No.	Various possibilities of drugs	Reference from various (source) books	Final suggestions Abbreviation of drug recommended and full name
1	2	3	4	5	6
1.	sol.	MIND—Excitable, p. 200	Sol. (Sun light) Solanium Solanum Aceticum Solanum arrebenta Solanum Carolinense Solanum lycopersicum Solanum mammosum Solanum nigrum Solanum oleraceum Solanum pseudo capsicum Solanum tuberosum aegrotanus	sun light C.M.M. Vol. III p. 1202 Mind—excitement and anxiousness in all her nerves, at first with trembling at heart, finally it remained in stomachpit; all that night and next day very sensitive and easily frightened;	Sol. (Sun light)
2.	amy.	MIND—AGGRAVATION Climacteric: p.223	Amygdalae-amarae-aqua. Amyl nitrite	Amyl nitrite Boe. p. 47 Palpitation of the heart and Similar conditions are readily cured by it, especially the flushing and other discomforts at climacteric	Amy. - n. Amyl nitrite

112

1	2	3	4	5	6
3.	Amy.	SENSORIUM—confusion vertex: p.236	Amygdalae-amarae-aqua amyl nitrite	Amyl nitrite A.E. Vol. I, p. 309 HEAD - consufion of head. After the throbbing and fullness of the head had passed away, it was followed by a confused weak feeling and a weight in top of head, as though it would be crushed in; — Sensation of something rushing upwards and throbbing in vertex.	Amy-n. Amyl nitrite
4.	lad-c.	VERTIGO—AMELIORATION—Sitting, up in bed: p. 247	Lac caninum Lac vaccinum defloratum	Lac vaccinum defloratum C.M.M. Vol. II, p. 206, Vertigo: on moving head from pillow; < lying down and especially turning while lying, obliging to sit up.	Lac-v-d. Lac vaccinum defloratum
5.	Mer.	HEAD—Internal—middle of : p. 251	Mercurialis perennis	Mercurialis perennis A. E. Vol. VI. p. 195. Pressure in the forehead & sinciput, in the region of the glabella and root of the nose (after 1½ hours).	Merl. Mercurialis perennis
6.	Org.	HEAD—INTERNAL—Ears, extending to : p. 262	Oreodaphne Origanum Origanum majorana Ornithogalum	Oreodaphne Boe. p. 489 HEAD – constant, dull ache in cervical and occipital region; extending to scapula down spine, into the head, pain into the ears.	Ore. Oreodaphne

1	2	3	4	5	6
7.	Amy.	HEAD—INTERNAL AGGRAVATION Climacteric: p. 282	*Amygdalae amarea aqua* *Amyl nitrite*	Amyl nitric Boe. p. 47 Surging of blood to head and face; — sensation as if blood would start through skin, with heat and redness. Flushing, following by sweat at climacteric	Amy-n. Amyl nitrite
8.	Am-b.	HEAD—INTERNAL—AGGRAVATION Dinner, after p. 238	*Ambra grisea* *Ambrosia artemisiae folia* *Ammonium benzoicum* *Ammonium bromatum* *Ammonium carbonicum*	Ambra grisea A.E. Vol. I p. 239 Head — oppressive confusion of the head, immediately after eating	Ambr. Ambra grisea
9.	mgs.	EYES—CANTHI—itching—outer: p. 332	*Magnesia sulphurica* *Mezereum*	Mezereum A. E. Vol. VI, p. 386 Itching in the right external canthus and agglutination as from mucus, very disagreeable obliging him to wipe and rub without relief.	Mez. Mezereum
10.	Mang-p.	TEETH AGGRAVATION bed in: 434	*Magnesia phosphorica*	Magnesia phosphorica H.G.S. Vol. VII p. 250 Toothache, teeth sensitive agg. After going on bed.	Mag-phos. Magnesia phosphorica
11.	Meg.	TEETH—CONCOMITANTS blood, rushes of : p. 439	*Mezereum*	Mezereum C.M.M. Vol. II, p. 486 TEETH Ebullition of blood to the head, shivering and constipation, during toothaches.	Mez. Mezereum

1	2	3	4	5	6
12.	Crp.	MOUTH TONGUE.— Tongue: p. 462	*Cuprum metallicum*	Cuprum metallicum C.M.M. Vol. I. P. 641 MOUTH-TONGUE, Clammy, loaded with a white coating	Cupr. Cuprum metallicum
13.	Chin-r.	MOUTH—TIME Night: p. 469	*Cinnabaris*	Cinnabaris H.G.S. Vol. IV p. 205 Inflammation with dryness in mouth and throat, < at night which cause him to drink often.	Cinnb. Cinnabaris
14.	arn-t.	MOUTH— AGGRAVATION— Coughing: p. 470	*Arum triphyllum*	Arum triphyllum H.G.S. Vol. II. p. 175 COUGH—Frequent coughing with much mucus and much spitting	Arum-t. Arum triphyllum
15.	Dull.	Mouth—AGGRAVATION— Speaking p. 471	*Dulcamara*	**Dulcamara** Ch. Dis. Vol. I p. 697 Paralysis of the tongue interfering with speaking (in cold damp weather)	Dulc. Dulcamara
16.	Cast-r.	APPETITE—Desire warm or hot drinks: p.477	*Castanea vesca*	Castanea vesca Boe. p. 179— Desire for warm drinks	Cast-v. Castanea vesca
17.	Stro.	TASTE—Earthy: p. 484	*Strontium* *Strophanthus hispidus*	Strontium C.M.M. Vol III p. 1284 Appetite—Earthy Taste in mouth	Stront. Strontium

1	2	3	4	5	6
18.	gell.	TASTE—spoiled; p. 488	Gelsemium sempervirens	Gelsemium sempervirens Boenninghausen's Repertory p. 69 MOUTH— TASTE — foul, spoiled taste	Gels. Gelsemium sempervirens
19.	dulI.	WATER BRASH AND HEART BURN—hot. p. 496	Dulcamara	Dulcamara Ch. Dis. p. 697-98 Sensation of increased warmth in the fauces – vomiting of mucus, in the morning, after previous warm rising in the fauces.	Dulc. Dulcamara
20.	mrl.	WATER BRASH AND HEART BURN—agg. Stopping: p. 498	Mercurialis perennis	Mercurialis perennis A.E. Vol. VI. p. 200 Stomach– Violent eructation, especially on stooping– Eructation tasting of the drug (after an hour) eructation of a horribly bitter, billious taste (first to 3 days). Water brash (after 6 and 20 hours).	Merl. Mercurialis perennis
21.	mag-n.	HICCOUGH Hiccough:— p. 498	Magnesia phosphorica	Magnesia phosphorica Boe. p. 417 STOMACH– Hiccough with retching day and night	Mag-p. Magnesia phosphorica
22.	Merc-cl.	NAUSEA AND VOMITTING Purging with: p. 504	Mercurius dulcis	Mercurius dulcis A.E. Vol. VI, p. 268 Stomach — profuse vomiting and diarrhea	Merc-d Mercurius dulcis

1	2	3	4	5	6
23.	Stro.	STOMACH—Squeezing in: p. 520	*Strontium* Strophanthus hispidus	Strontium H.G.S. Vol. X., p. 91 Scrobiculum and Stomach Constriction in stomach, with uprisings of clear water.	Stront. Strontium
24.	Sp-u-di	STOMACH AND EPIGASTRIUM AGG.— Salt, abuse of: p. 529	*Nitri Spiritus dulcis*	Nitri Spiritus dulcis H.G.S. Vol. VIII, p. 44 Scrobiculum and Stomach. Aching, contracting pain from eating too much salt.	Nit-s-d. Niotri Spiritus dulcis
25.	atp-s.	HYPOCHONDRIA— pancreas: p. 534	*Atropinium sulphuricum*	Atropinum sulphuricum H.G.S. Vol. II, p. 262 Vomiting appears sometimes in evening between 6 and 7; then in night between 11 and 1 o'clock, regularly 5, 6 hours after a full meal. Q diseased pancreas.	Atro. Atropinnium sulphuricum
26.	Chan.	ABDOMEN—AGG. Respiratory symptoms during: p. 563	*Chamomilla*	Chamomilla C.M.M. Vol. I, p. 458 Burning cutting in epigastrium, with difficulty of respiration and paleness of the face.	Cham. Chamomilla
27.	Stro.	ABDOMEN- AGG. Turning the body : p. 564	*Strontium* Strophanthus hispidus	Strontium H.G.S. Vol. X, p. 91 Scrobiculum and stomach – pressure in pit of stomach, aching in stomach; > by eating; > on walking.	Stront. Strontium

1	2	3	4	5	6
28.	tap.	FLATULENCE–AGG. Inspiration: p. 580	*Staphysagria*	Staphysargria 1 M.M. Pura Vol. II p. 567 Transient pressive pain as from displaced fluctulence under rib. A contraction in the hypochondria oppressing the chest and impending respiration.	Staph. Staphysagrie
29.	ant-s-n.	STOOL– CONSTIPATION– aged of the: p. 583	*Antimonium sulphuratum aureum*	Antimonium sulphuratum aureum C.M.M. Vol. I, p. 127-28 Clinical-constipation stool-constipations feces hard and passed with difficulty.	Ant-s. Antimonium sulphuratum aureum
30.	Uran-n	STOOL CONSTIPATION Colic, flatulent, with: p. 584	*Uranium nitricum*	Uranium nitgricum C.M.M. Vol. III. p. 1478 Abdomen.– Borborygmi. Sharp colic, with tenesmus and with raw feeling in rectum.	Uran-n. Uranium nitricum
31.	Chell.	STOOL DIARRHEA– painless: p. 585	*Chelidonium majus*	Chelidcnium majus H.G.S. Vol. IV, p. 19 Diarrhea without pain, without urging.	Chel. Chelidonium majus
32.	mag-a	STOOL-CONCOMITANTS BEFORE STOOL ABDOMEN rumbling etc. in: p. 593	*Magnesia carbonica*	Magnesia carbonica C.M.M. Vol. II, p. 361 Gripping, cutting and rumbling in whole abdomen followed by thin green stool, without tenesmus.	Mag-c. Magnesia carbonica

1	2	3	4	5	6
33.	Sacc.	STOOL CONCOMITANT BEFORE STOOL odor of body; p. 594	Saccharum lactis Saccharum album	Saccharum lactis, C.M.M. Vol. III p. 1057 before stool hands and whole body exhaled a fecal odor, which passed away after stool.	Sacc. l. Saccharum lactis
34.	mag-ac	STOOL-CONCOMITANTS, BEFORE-STOOL-Abdomen-griping, colic etc. in: 593	Magnetis polus Arcticus	Magnetis polus arcticus H.C. Allen Nosodes p. 232 Stool – Drawing almost dysenteric pain in the hypogastrium early in morning followed by difficult expulsion of the very thick feces	Mag-arct. Magnetis polus Arcticus
35.	Ura.	URINE-ODOR-Fishbrine, like: p. 621	Uranium nitricum	Uranium nitricum H.G.S. Vol. X. p. 360 Urine greenish and smelling fishy.	Uran. Uranium nitricum
36.	Chimp.	URINE-SEDIMENT-Adherent: p. 623	Chimaphila maculata Chimaphila umbellata	Chimaphila umbellate H.G.S. Vol. IV, p. 57 Urine high colored, depositing a copious mucus sediment dysuria	Chim. Chimaphila umbellata
37.	Chimp.	URINE-SEDIMENT-Gelatinous; p. 624	Chimaphila umbellata Chimaphila maculata	Chimaphila umbellate C.M.M. Vol. I, p. 475. URINARY– organs Great quantities of think, ropy blood mucus in urine.	Chim. Chimaphila umbellata

1	2	3	4	5	6
38.	am-b.	URINE—SEDIMENT—Sandy (gravelly): p. 624	Ambra grisea, Ambrosia Artemisiae folia Ammonium benzoicum Ammonium bromatum Ammonium cabonicum	Ambra grisea, C.M.M. Vol. I, p. 77 Urinary organs-urine of yellowish-brown, and turbid, with brown sediment.	Ambr. Ambra grisea
39.	Chimp	URINE—SEDIMENT—Slimy, mucus: p. 624	Chimaphila umbellata Chimaphila maculata	Chimaphila umbellata H.G.S. Vol. IV, p. 57, Scanty urine, with muco-purulent sediments.	Chim Chimaphila umbellata
40.	aur-t.	URINE MICTURITION—urination Profuse, copious, polyuria, etc.: p. 627	Arum t:iphyllum	Arum triphyllum C.M.M. Vol. I, p. 201 URINARY—ORGANS—Frequent discharge of abundant pale urine – clear, watery urine and smelling like burnt horn.	Arum-t. Arum triphyllum
41.	Chimap	URINE-BEFORE URINATION-Labor like Pain: p. 630	Chimaphila umbellata Chimaphila maculata	Chimaphila umbellata F.M.M. p. 92 – It produces frequent urination at night debility and smarting pain extending from the neck of the bladder to the end of the urethra	Chim. Chimaphila umbellata
42.	berg.	URINE-BEFORE URINATION-urethra burning in: p. 630	Berberis vulgaris	Berberis vulgaris Boe. p. 120 URINARY– urethra burns when not urinating.	Berb. Berberis vulgaris

1	2	3	4	5	6
43.	arum	URINARY ORGANS— KIDNEYS –Burning heat etc. in: p. 637	*Aurum dracontium* *Arum italicum* *Arum maculatum* *Arum triphyllum*	Aurum dracontium Boe. p. 87 – URINARY – burns and smarts.	Arum-d. Aurum dracontium
44.	tellur.	URINARY ORGANS— KIDNEYS Heaviness: p. 638	*Tellurium*	Tellurium C.M.M. Vol. III. p. 1388 Female sexual organs Painful soreness in region of kidneys extending downward like a weight, mostly to right and in sacrum	Tell. Tellurium
45.	Cimb.	URINARY ORGANS URETHRA Discharge Yellow green : p. 642	*Cinnabaris* *Cinnamomum*	Cinnabaris H.G.S. Vol. IV, p. 207 MALE sexual organs yellowish green discharge	Cinnb. Cinnabaris
46.	Cimb.	GENITALIA–MALE– ORGANS–Figwarts, condylomata: p. 646	*Cinnabaris* *Cinnamomum*	Cinnabaris C.M.M. Vol. I, p. 528– Male– sexual organs condyloma; sycotic excrescences.	Cinnb. Cinnabaris
47.	Cimb.	GENITALIA–PENIS Swelling : p. 649	*Cinnabaris* *Cinnamomum*	Cinnabaris C.M.M. Vol. I. p. 528 Male – Sexual– organs: swelling of the penis	Cinnab. Cinnabaris
48.	Cinb.	GENITALIA– GLANS GLANS: p. 649	*Cinnabaris* *Cinnamomum*	Cinnabaris C.M.M. Vol. I, p. 528 MALE – Sexual – organs – small, shining red points on the glans penis.	Cinnb. Cinnabaris

1	2	3	4	5	6
49.	Can.	GENITALIA–glans moisture: p. 650	Cannabis indica Cannabis sativa	Cannabis sativa T.F. Allen p. 264 Moisture about corona glands – Prepuce – itching beneath, prepuce and on forenum, with redness and moisture behind corona glands.	Cann-s. Cannabis sativa
50.	Cimb.	GENITALIA–Glans moisture: p. 50	Cinnabaris Cinnamomum	Cinnabaris A.E. Vol. III, p. 328 Two small red spots appeared on each side of the glans, secreting a large quantity of lardaceous matter T.F. Allen – 254 – Moisture about corona glandis.	Cinnb. Cinnabaris
51.	Can.	GENITALIA–PREPUCE – Redness : p. 651	Cannabis indica Cannabis sativa	Cannabis sativa A.E. Vol. II, p. 499 The whole prepuce is dark red, hot and inflamed.	Cann-s. Cannabis sativa
52.	Cimb.	GENITALIA–PREPUCE– Redness: p. 651	Cinnabaris Cinnamomum	Cinnabaris A.E. Vol. II, p. 327 MALE – Redness and swelling of the prepuce	Cinnb. Cinnabaris
53.	Can.	GENITALIA– Prepuce– Swelling: p. 652	Cannabis indica Cannabis sativa	Cannabis sativa A.E. Vol. II, p. 499 Swelling of the right side and lower portion of the prepuce.	Cann-s. Cannabis sativa

1	2	3	4	5	6
			Cinnabaris *Cinnamonum*	Cinnabaris A.E. Vol. III, p. 327 – MALE Redness and swelling of the prepuce.	Cinnb. Cinnabaris
54.	Cimb.	GENITALIA–Prepuce–Swelling: p. 652			
55.	aur-p.	GENITALIA TESTES–Hard: p. 653.	*Aurum metallicum*	Aurum metallicum T.F. Allen p. 154 Testes swollen and hard (Rhod., Puls.)	Aur. Aurum metallicum
56.	mex.	GENITALIA FEMALE Organs–dryness vagina: p. 659	*Murex purpurea*	Murex purpurea C.M.M. Vol. II, p. 507 Female sexual organs sensation of dryness, and contraction of uterus.	Murx. Murex purpurea
57.	Deph.	SEXUAL IMPUSE–Erection, toothache, during: p. 670	*Daphne Indica*	Dephne indica C.M.M. Vol. I p. 657, MALE SEXUAL ORGANS–Erection during the toothache–toothache after coition.	Daph. Daphne indica
58.	Deph.	SEXUAL IMPUSE–Prostatic fluid, loss of: p. 671	*Daphne Indica*	Daphne indica C.M.M. Vol. I, p. 657, MALE SEXUAL ORGANS – Discharge of Prostate fluid	Daph. Daphne Indica
59.	Stro.	MENSTRUATION–Menstrual – blood pale: p. 677.	*Strontium*	Strontium C.M.M. Vol. III, p. 1284 Female sexual organs – Retarded catamenia, at first serous (like meat water), afterwards in clots.	Stront. Strontium

1	2	3	4	5	6
60.	Amy.	MENSTRUATION–CONCOMITANTS BEFORE MENSES Uterus: p. 679	Amygdalae amarae aqua Amyl nitrite	Amyl nitrite Boe. p. 48 Female. After pains; hemorrhage associated with facial flushing.	Amyl-n. Amyl nitrite
61.	Ur-n.	MENSTRUATION–CONCOMITANTS DURING MENSES–SENSORIUM Faintness: p. 682	Uranium nitricum	Uranium nitricum H.G.S. Vol. X. p. 360 Female sexual organs. During menstruation: vertigo; faint; flushing of upper part of body.	Uran Uranium nitricum
62.	Carb-b.	RESPIRATION–IMPEDED by–Breath, as if from want of : p. 695	Carboneum hydrogenisatum Carbo vegetabilis	Carbo vegetabilis Boger p. 157 Icy, but wants air.	Carb-v. Carbo vegetabilis
63.	Sp-n-d	COUGH–EXCITED or AGG. by LARYNX. Sticking in: p. 713	Spigelia marilandica Spigelia anthelmintica	Spigelia anthelmintica, T.F. Allen p. 1028 stitching in region of Larynx... hollow cough.	spig. Spigelia anthelmintica
64.	Saes	COUGH–CONCOMITANTS–Throat Roughness in: p. 726	Sarsaparilla	Sarsaparilla K.P. 802 COUGH – Roughness in larynx causes cough	Sars. Sarsaparilla
65.	Croc-c.	COUGH–CONCOMITANTS–Vomiting: p. 726	Cocculus indicus Coccinella—septempunctata, Coccus cacti.	Coccus cacti. Boger p. 174. Racking – cough – ending into vomiting	Coc-c. Coccus cacti.

1	2	3	4	5	6
			Angustura vera.	Angustura vera K.P. 819 Expectoration – Taste salty	Ang. Angustura vera
66.	amg.	COUGH–EXPECTORATION Taste of salty : p. 733			
67.	Ver-b.	NECK AND EXTERNAL THROAT, NAPE head, ascending into: p. 749	Veratrum album Veratrum viride	Veratrum viride H.G.S. Vol. X, 425 Headache from nape of neck with vertigo, dim vision.	Verat-v. Veratrum viride
68.	tap.	CHEST INNER–RIBS, between, Intercostal: p. 754	Staphysagria	Staphysagria Kent, p. 861 CHEST PAIN Costal cartilages	Staph. Staphysagria
69.	Seng.	CHEST INNER PRESSURE load or weight, as of a : p. 759	Senega	Senega C.M.M. Vol. III, p. 1156 Pressure in chest Boe p. 585 Respiratory – much mucus; sensation of oppression and weight of chest.	Seneg. Senega
70.	Can.	CHEST INNER Quivering internal; p. 760	Cannabis indica Cannabis sativa	Cannabis sativa M.M. Pura Vol. I, p. 321 Quivering as of in the blood of the head, chest and stomach.	Cann-s. Cannabis sativa
71.	Chena	BACK SCAPULAR REGION– Scapulae, right: p. 785	Chenopodium anthelminticum Chenopodium vulvaria Chenopodium glauciaphis	Chenopodium anthelminticum Boe. p. 191 BACK—intense pain between angle of right shoulder blade—near spine, and through the chest.	Chen-a. Chenopodium anthelminticum

1	2	3	4	5	6
72.	Chena	BACK, SCAPULAR REGION– Scapulae, left: p. 785	*Chenopodium anthelminticum Chenopodi glauci aphis Chenopodium vulvaria Chenopodium glauciaphis*	Chenopodi glauci aphis Boe. p. 192 Back—severe pains in region of lower inner angle of left shoulder—blade, running into chest.	Chen. Chenopodi Glauci aphis
73.	Chena.	BACK, SCAPULAR Region– left: angle, of: p. 785	*Chenopodium anthelminticum, Chenopodi glauci, aphis, Chenopodium vulvaria*	Chenopodi glauci aphis same as sl. no. 72	Chen Chenopodi Glauci aphis
74.	Calac.	BACK LUMBAR REGION SMALL OF BACK IN GENERAL— Lumbar (also loins) p. 793	*Calcarea carbonica Hahnemanni Calcarea acetica Calcarea arsenica*	Calcarea acetica T.F. Allen p. 234 soreness between nates when walking Heart and back cutting, pressing out pain in right loin.	Calc-ac. Calcarea acetica
75.	Agaf.	BACK–BACK PROPER– DORSAL REGION Tension p. 792	*Asafoetida*	Asafoetida C.M.M. Vol. I. p. 206 NECK & BACK – cannot work on account of the backache.	Asaf. Asafoetida
76.	Berb.	BACK–LUMBAR REGION– SMALL OF BACK IN GENERAL Burning: p. 793	*Berberis vulgaris*	Berberis vulgaris KP 919 BACK LUMBAR PAIN – Burning.	Berb. Berberis vulgaris

1	2	3	4	5	6
77.	arg-n.	BACK–LUMBAR REGION SMALL OF BACK IN GENERAL—Heaviness, load, etc.: p. 794	*Argentum nitricum*	Argentum nitricum K.P. 891 BACK – HEAVINESS Lumbar region	Arg-n. Argentum nitricum
78.	Can.	LOWER EXTREMITIES– Loins, (Hip) region, p. 842	*Cannabis indica* *Cannabis sativa*	Cannabis indica C.M.M. Vol. I, p. 380 lower limbs on attempting to walk; intensely violent pain as if treading on spikes, which penetrated the soles, and ran upward through the limbs on the hips; worse in r. limb, and accompanied by drawing pains in both calves.	Cann-I. Cannabis indica
79.	Stro.	LOWER EXTREMITIES– Weak and weary: p. 873	*Strontium strophanthus hispidus*	Strontium H.G.S. Vol. X, p. 92 limbs in general great emaciation.	Stront. Strontium
80.	muc-ac.	SENSATION AND COMPLAINTS IN GENERAL– Constriction (Contraction) sense of, of external parts: p. 888	*Muriaticum acidum*	Muriaticum acidum K.P. 966 EXTREMITIES CONTRACTION of muscles and tendons.	Mur-ac. Muriaticum acidum

1	2	3	4	5	6
81.	Vio.	SENSATION AND COMPLAINTS IN GENERAL—Constriction (Contraction) sense of, external parts: p. 888	Viola odorata	Viola odorata H.G.S. Vol. X p. 476 Sensation – burning like a small transient flame in spots here and there	Viol-o. Viola odorata
82.	m-arct.	SENSATION AND COMPLAINTS IN GENERAL—Cramp, in joints: p. 890	Magnetis polus Arcticus	Magnetis polus Arcticus H.C. Allen Nosodes p. 234 Upper Extremities– Cramp- Like sensation in arms, and as if it had gone to sleep.	Mag-p-a. Magnetis polus australis
83.	verb-v.	SENSATION AND COMPLAINTS IN GENERAL– Fungoid growth: p. 899	Berberis vulgaris	Berberis vulgaris Boe p. 181 circumscribed pigmentation following eczematous inflammation	Berb-v. Berberis vulgaris
84.	Croc.	SENSATION AND COMPLAINTS IN GENERAL—Hemorrhages, tenacious, stringy, etc.: p. 901	Crocus sativus	Crocus sativus H.G.S. Vol. IV p. 477 FEMALE sexual organs menses– blood dark, clotted, and stringly, v scid.	Croc-s. Crocus sativus
85.	Mang.	SENSATION AND COMPLAINTS IN GENERAL– piercing, boring, grinding, grating: p. 913.	Magnesia carbonica Magnesia phosphorica Magnesia muriatica Magnesia sulphurica	Magnesic phosphorica H.G.S. Vol. VII, p. 255 SENSATION Piercing all over him agg. about ankles, knees, and elbows	Mag-phos. Magnesia phosphorica

1	2	3	4	5	6
86.	Cimb.	SENSATION AND COMPLAINTS IN GENERAL– Slide, left: p. 920	*Cinnabaris*	Cinnabaris C.M.M. Vol. I. p. 529 Upper limbs– numbness of left arm, from elbow to end of little finger, it feel as if the crazy– bone was struck.	Cinnb. Cinnabaris
87.	HY-p.	SENSATION AND COMPLAINTS IN GENERAL – spasms tonic: p. 922	*Hypericum perforatum*	Hypericum perforatum K.P. 968 Extremities convulsions A.E. Vol. V. p. 58 Inferior extremities foot– cramp in left foot knee, Transient cramp in the knee. Superior extremities – Trembling and cramp in left arm and fingers H.G.S. Vol. VI. p. 117 Sensorium – with feeling of weakness and trembling of limbs.	Hyp. Hypericum perforatum
88.	hip.	SENSATION AND COMPLAINTS IN GENERAL–starting as in affright: p. 924	*Hippomanes*	Hippomanes A.E. Vol. IV. p. 594 Weakness of the arms and limbs at first for one day – weakness and weariness in the limbs.	Hipp. Hippomanes
89.	Turb	SENSATION AND COMPLAINTS IN GENERAL– stopped gait: p. 926	*Terebinthinaes oleum*	Terebinthinaes oleum C.M.M. Vol. III. p. 1399. Heaviness of limbs, sensation of stiffness in all muscles, with difficult, slow stooping gait, as in old age.	Ter. Terebinthinae oleum

1	2	3	4	5	6
90.	sen-ac	SENSATION AND COMPLAINTS IN GENERAL– Stretching twist, inclined to, drawing up and stretching out alternatively: p. 926	*Senecio aureus*	Senecio aureus C.M.M. Vol. III p. –1150 Lower limbs– constant desire to keep feet in motion.	Senec. Senecio aureus
91.	Calclyp.	SENSATION AND COMPLAINTS IN GENERAL– Suppuration: p. 926	*Calcarea hypophosporosa*	Calcarea hypophosporosa Boe. p. 153 (is to be preferred when it seems necessary to furnish the organism with liberal doses of phosphorus in consequence continued abscesses– having reduced the vitality.	Calcar. hypophosporosa
92.	pyso.	SENSATION AND COMPLAINTS IN GENERAL– Tossing about (in bed) : p. 931	*Pyrogenium*	Pyrogenium H.C. Allen Nosodes p. 420. Automatic movement for r.arm r. leg, turned the child round from r. to l till feet reached the pillow; repeated as often as she was put right (ceerebrospinal meningitis).	Pyrog. Pyrogenium
93.	cut-h	SENSATION AND COMPLAINTS IN GENERAL– Trembling, shaking sense of internal: p. 932	*Crotalus horridus*	Crotalus horridus C.M.M. Vol. I. p. 617 lower limbs trembling	Crot-h. Crotalus horridus

1	2	3	4	5	6
94.	senio	SENSATION AND COMPLAINTS IN GENERAL– waves undulations: p. 934	Senecio aureus	Senecio aureus Boe. p. 583 Head wave like dizziness from occiput to sinciput.	Senec. Senecio aureus
95.	ars-s.	GLANDS– Swelling (tumour): p. 939	Arsenicum iodatum	Arsenicum iodatum Boe. p. 85 Enlargment scrofulous glands	Ars. i. Arsenicum iodatum
96.	sulforal	SKIN AND EXTERIOR BODY – Eruption, measly; p. 951	Sulphur	Sulphur C.M.M. Vol. III p. p. 1299 Clinical – measles	Sulph. Sulphur
97.	eucl	SLEEP CHARACTER OF – weakness with: p. 986	Eucalyptus globules	Eucalyptus globules A.E.Vol. IV. p. 230 sleep– feel sleepy and dull drowsiness in anemic subject.	Eucal. Eucalyptus globulus
98.	pys.	DREAMS–DAY'S WORK, events of the day; p. 999	Pyrogenium	Pyrogenium H.C. Allen Nosode p. 422 Dreamed all night of the busines of the day	Pyrog. Pyrogenium
99.	chan	FEVER PATHOLOGICAL TYPES– Scarlet fever, irregular p. 1004	Chamomilla	Chamomilla A.E. Vol. III. p. 124 Fever heat... very profuse sweat on the feet	Cham. Chamomilla

1	2	3	4	5	6
100.	cups	CIRCULATION CONGESTION— Stagnated feeling, obstructed as if p. 1010	Cuprum sulphuricum	Cuprum sulphuricum H.G.S. Vol. V., p. 51 Heart pulse circulation— Feeling as of throbbing lump in heart, internally beating of heart seemed louder, lasted five minutes and went away gradually.	Cup-s Cuprum sulphuricum
101.	stup	CIRCULATION PALPITATION — Palpitation, in general page 1010	Sticta pulmonaria	Sticta pulmonaria H.G.S. Vol. X p. 32 Attacks of great anxiety about heart, very nervous; had had much mental trouble; awake at night with a strange sensation about heart, and for a few moments aftrer feels as if she were floating in air.	Stict. Sticta pulmonaria
102.	vio-v.	CIRCULATION— PALPITATION— violent Page 1012	Viola odorata	Viola odorata AE Vol. X, p. 132 Respiratory organs— Associated with violent beating of the heart.	Viol-o. Viola odorata
103.	pyng	CIRCULATION-PULSE pulse, abnormal in general: p. 1014	Pyrogenium	Pyrogenium H.C. Allen Nosodes p. 419 loud, heartbeats audible to herself and others.	Pyrog. Pyrogenium

132

1	2	3	4	5	6
104.	mag-n.	FEVER–PARTIAL COLDNESS– partial coldness, Head–forehead: p. 1025	*Manganum*	Manganum C.M.M., Vol. II p. 406 FEVER– chill with heat of head stinging pain in forehead which continues after the chill.	Mang. Manganum
105.	Spire	FEVER–SENSE of partial coldness– partical throat in: p. 1028	*Spiranthes*	Spiranthes C.M.M. Vol. III p. 1236 FEVER– Alternation of cold and heat, affected part colder than rest of body.	Spira Spiranthes
106.	polyp-o.	FEVER–SENSE OF PARTIAL COLDNESS– partial back. spine: p. 1029	*Polyporus Offcinalis*	Polyporus officinalis H.G.S. Vol. VIII p. 530 Fever– chills creeping along spine.– Frequent creeping chills along spine.	Poly-o. Polyporus officinalis
107.	Caun	HEAD AND FEVER IN GENERAL – PARTIAL heat – on plate: p. 1053	*Caulophyllum Thalictroides*	Caulophyllum Thalictrides H.G.S. Vol. III p. 428 INNER– MOUTH sensation of dryness in mouth; heat.	Caul. Caulophyllum Thalictroides
108.	Carb-m	AGGRAVATION AND AMELIORATION IN GENERAL vaulted places, damp cellars vaults, agg:: p. 1148	*Carduus marianus*	Carduus marianus Boger p. 158 < cellars	Card-m. Carduus marianus

APPENDIX - A

BOOKS IN ENCYCLOPEDIA (RADAR) HOMEOPATHICA SOFTWARE

Type indicates the focus of the document:

CA	—	Cases
CL	—	Clinical Information
JO	—	Journal
MM	—	Materia Medica
PH	—	Philosophy
PR	—	Provings
RE	—	Repertory Extractions
TH	—	Therapeutics

Author	Book/Title	Type
Allen H.C.	The Therapeutics of Intermittent Fever	MM
”	The Materia Medica with the Nosodes and Provings of X-ray	MM
”	Keynotes and Characteristics with Comparisons	MM
Allen John H.	The Chronic Miasms, Psora & Pseudopsora	PH
Allen T.F.	Handbook of Materia Medica and Homeopathic Therapeutics	MM
”	Encyclopedia of Pure Materia Medica (10 vols.)	MM

"	A Primer of Materia Medica	MM
American Homeopath	1995-2001	JO
American Institute of Homeopathy, Journal of the	1935	JO
American Institute of Homeopathy, Transactions of the 16th Session	1904	JO
Anonymous Author	The Poultry Doctor	MM
Anshutz E.P.	Sexual Ills and Diseases	TH
"	New, Old and Forgotten Remedies	MM
Baehr Bernhard	The Science of Therapeutics, According to The Principle of Homeopathy Vol. I	PH
"	The Science of Therapeutics, According to The Principles of Homeopathy Vol. II	PH
Benerjee P.	Materia Medica of Indian Drugs	MM
Banerjee P. N.	Chronic Diseases, its Cause and Cure	
Banerjee S. K.	Materia Medica Made Easy	
"	Fifty Homeopathic, Indian Drugs	MM

"	Materia Medica of a Few Rare Remedies (Lyss., Morb., Sanic. Strptoc. Staphycoc. Thyr.)	PR
Bedayn Greg	Corvus corax	PR
Bell J. B.	The Homeopathic Therapeutics of Diarrhea	MM
Benson A. Reuel	Homeopathic Nursery Manual	TH
Berjaeau J.P.H. & Frost J.H.P.	Homeopathic Treatment of Syphilis, Gonorrhea Spermatorrhea and Urinary Diseases	TH
Bernard H.	The Homeopathic Treatment of Constipation	TH
Bhatia V. R.	Influenza and Its Homeopathic Treatment	TH
Bidwell Glen Irving	How to Use the Repertory with a Practical Analysis of Forty Homeopathic Remedies	PH
Blackie Margery G.	A Comparison of Ars. Nit. Acid., Hep., Sulph. and Nux vomica	MM
Blackwood A. L.	The food Tract; its Ailments and Disease of the Peritoneum	TH
"	Disease of the Liver, Pancreas and Ductless Glands	TH
"	Diseases of the Kidneys and Nerves	TH

"	Diseases of the Heart	TH
"	A Manual of Materia Medica Therapeutics and Pharmacology with	MM
Boericke W.	Clinical Index	MM
Boenninghausen Clemens Von	The Twelve Tissue Remedies of Schussler	PH
Boericke W.	The Lesser Writings	MM
Boger C. M.	Pocket Manual of Homeopathic Materia Medica	PH
"	The Study of Materia Medica and Case Taking	MM
"	Synoptic Key of the Materia Medica	MM
Bond Annette	Boenninghausen's Characterstics and Repertory	PR
Bonnerot	The Homeopathic Proving of Tungsten	TH
Borland D. M.	Ulcer of Stomach and Duodenum	PH
"	The Treatment of Certain Heart Conditions	TH
"	Some Emergencies of General Practice	TH
"	Pneumonia	MM
"	Influenzas	MM

"	Homeopathy in Practice	MM
"	Homeopathy for Mother and Infant	TH
"	Digestive Drugs	TH
"	Children Types	TH
Bouko Levy M.M.	Homeopathic and Drainage Repertory	TH
Bradford Thomas Lindsley	Index of Homeopathic Provings	PH
"	The Life and Letters of Hahnemann	PH
The British Homeopathic Journal	1911-1913	JO
Buck H.	The Outlines of Materia Medica and a Clinical Dictionary	MM
The Bureau of Homeopathics	1924	JO
Burnett J. C.	Ringworm	PR
"	Vaccinosis	CA
"	Tumours of the Breasts	CA
"	The New Cure for Consumption by Its Own Virus	CA

"	The Disease of the Liver	MM
"	The Change of Life in Women and the Ills and Ailings Incident Thereto	PH
"	Organ Diseases of Women	CA
"	On Neuralgia	CA
"	On Fistula and Its Radical Cure by Medicines	TH
"	Natrum Muriaticum	CA
"	Gout and Its Cure	MM
"	Gold as a Remedy in Disease Notable in some forms of Organic Heart Disease, Angina Pectoris, Melancholy…	CA
"	and as an Antidote to the Effects of Mercury	CA
"	Fifty Reasons for Being a Homeopath	TH
"	Fevers and Blood Poisoning	TH
"	Enlarged Tonsils Cured by Medicine	TH
"	Diseases of the Spleen	CA
"	Diseases of the Skin	CA
"	Delicate, Backward, Puny and Stunty Children	CA

	Curability of Tumours by Medicines	TH
	Curability of Cataract	TH
Burt W. H.	Characteristic Materia Medica	MM
"	Physiological Materia Medica	MM
Candegabe E. F.	Comparative Materia Medica	MM
Case Erastus	Some Clinical Experiences	MM
Castro Miranda	Borax veneta	MM
Central Council For Research In Homeopathy, New Delhi	A Proving of Cassia Sophera	PR
Chatterjee T. P.	My Random Notes on Some Homeo- Remedies	MM
"	My Memorable Cures	TH
"	Hints on Homeopathic Practice and Children's Disease	PH
"	Fundamentals of Homeopathy (Valuable Hints for Practice)	PH
Chatterji A. N.	Three in One	MM
Chauhan R. K.	Expressive Drug Pictures of Materia Medica Vol. 2	MM

"		Expressive Drug Pictures of Materia Medica Vol. 1	MM
Choudhuri N. M.		A Study on Materia Medica and Repertory	MM
Choudhury Harimohan		Indications of Miasm	TH
"		50 Millesimal Potency in Theory and Practice	MM
Clarke A. G.		Decachords	MM
Clarke J. H.		Bird's Eye View – A Lecture on Organon of Medicine	PH
"		The Cure of Tumours by Medicines	
"		Whooping Cough Cured with Coqueluchin	CA
Clarke J. H.		Therapeutics of Serpent Poison	MM
"		Therapeutics of Cancer	TH
"		The Prescriber	TH
"		Radium as an Internal Remedy	MM
"		Non-Surgical Treatment of Diseases of the Glands and Bones	TH
"		Indigestion - Its Cause and Cure	TH

”	Homeopathy Explained	PH
”	Hemorrhoids and Habitual Constipation: Their Constituitional Cure - with Chapters on Fissure and Fistula	TH
”		MM
”	Gunpowder as a War Remedy	MM
”	Grand Characteristics of Materia Medica	TH
”	Diseases of the Heart and Arteries	MM
”		CA
”	Dictionary of Practical Materia Medica (3 vols.)	TH
”	Constitutional Medicine, with Especial Reference of the Three Constitutions of Von Grauvogl	TH
"	Cholera, Diarrhea and Dysentery	TH
"	Catarrh, Colds and Influenza	TH
Cleveland C. L.	Salient Materia Medica and Therapeutics	MM
Close Stuart M.	The Genius of Homeopathy, Lectures and Essays on Homeopathic Philosophy	PH
Coulter Harris L.	Homeopathic Science and Modern Medicine. The Physics of Healing with Microdoses.	PH

Cowperthwaite A. C.	Textbook of Materia medica and Therapeutics	
Degroote F.	Physical Examination and Observation in Homeopathy	MM
Dewey W. A.	Practical Homeopathic Therapeutics	TH
"	Essentials of Homeopathic Materia Medica	MM
Digby B.	Lac caninum	MM
Douglass M. E.	Skin Diseases	TH
"	Pearls of Homeopathy	MM
"	Lectures on Theory and Practice of Homeopathy	PH
Duncan Thomas C.	Hand Book on the Disease of the Heart and Their Homeopathic Treatment	CL
Dunham Caroll	Lectures on Materia Medica	MM
"	The Science of Therapeutics: A Collection of Papers	PH
"	Symptoms, Their Study or "How to Take the Case"	PH
Eising Nuala	Ignis Alcoholis Succinum Provings (Fire)	PR

English Mary	Tempestas – Storm – A Remedy Proving	PR
Ennis Sylvia	Sickle Cell Disease / Thalassemia	TH
Epps John	Domestic Homeopathy: or, Rules for the Domestic Treatment of the Maladies of Infants, Children, and Adults, and for the Conduct and the Treatment During Pregnancy, Confinement, and Suckling. [5th Ed.]	TH
Farrington E. A.	Clinical Materia Medica	MM
"	Comparative Materia Medica (with Therapeutic Hints)	TH
"	Lesser Writing with Therapeutic Hints	TH
Fayazuddin M.	Hypericum – A Study (An Anti-Tetanus Remedy)	MM
"	Succus Calendula	MM
"	Surgeon's Friends in Homeopathy Arnica Montana	MM
Fisher C. E.	Homeopathy in Obstetric Emergencies	MM
Fortier-Bernoville	What We Must Not Do in Homeopathy	PH
"	Syphilis & Sycosis	
Foubister D. M.	The Carcinocin Drug Picture	MM

"	Significance of Past History in Homeopathic Prescribing	TH
"	Homeopathy and Paediatrics	TH
Gallavardin J. P.	Plastic Medicine Homeopathic Treatment	CA
"	Repertory of Psychic Medicines Materia Medica	MM
Gaskin A.	Comparative Study on Kent's Materia Medica	MM
Gentry William	Rubrical and Regional Text Book of Homeopathic Materia Medica Urine and Urinary Organs	CL
Geukens Aflons	Carcinosinum	RE
"	Homeopathic Practice Vol 6	CL
"	Homeopathic Practice Vol 5	CA
"	Homeopathic Practice Vol 4	CA
Geukens Alfons	Homeopathic Practice Vol 3	CA
"	Homeopathic Practice Vol 1	CA
"	Homeopathic Practice Vol 2	CA
Gibson D. M.	Studies of Homeopathic Remedies	MM

"	Elements of Homeopathy	PH
"	Fear and Homeopathy	
Gilchrist J. G.	The Homeopathic Treatment of Surgical Diseases	
Granier Michel	Conferences upon Homeopathy	CL
Grauvogl, Eduard Von	Text Book of Homeopathy Part 1 & 2	PH
Gray B. and Shore J.	Seminar Bur Haamstede April 1989	CA
Grimes Melanie	Tiger Shark: A Homeopathic Proving of Galeocerdo Cuvier Hepar	PR RE
Grimmer A. H. & Fortier-Bernoville	Homeopathic Treatment of Cancer (Ist Indian Ed.)	TH
Grimmer A. H.	The Collected Works	MM
Grinney Tony	A Proving of Thiosinamine	PR
Guanavante S. M.	The "Genius" of Homeopathic remedies	MM
Guernsey Egbert	Homeopathic Domestic Practice. [9th Ed.]	MM
Guernsey H. N.	Keynotes to the Materia Medica	MM

"	Application of Principles of Homeopathy to Obstertrics and the Disorders Peculiar to Young Children	TH
Guernsey W. J.	The Homeopathic Therapeutics of Haemorrhoids	MM
Gupta A. K.	The Problem Child and Homeopathy	TH
Gupta R. L.	Directory of Diseases and Cures in Homeopathy Vol 1 & Vol. 2	TH
Haehl Richard	Samuel Hahnemann: His Life and Work. Vol. 1	PH
"	Samuel Hahnemann: His life and Work Vol. 2	PH
Hahnemann S.	Organon	PH
"	Materia Medica Pura (2 vols.)	MM
"	Lesser writings Hahnemann	PH
"	Organon of the Medical Art by Dr. Samuel Hahnemann	PH
"		MM
"	Chronic Diseases (2 vols.)	
Hahnemannian Advocate	1896 – Volume XXXV	JO
"	1897 – Volume XXXVI	JO

"	1898 – Volume XXXVII	JO
The Hahnemannian Monthly	Vol 01 (08/1865 – 07/1866)	JO
"	Vol 07 (08/1871 – 07/1872)	JO
The Hahnemannian Monthly	Vol 08 – (08/1872 – 07/1873)	JO
"	Vol 24 – 1889 (01/02/03)	JO
"	Vol 25 – 1890 (05/06/10)	JO
"	Vol 32 – 1897 (03)	JO
"	June 1895	JO
Hale Edwin Moses	The Characteristics of the New Remedies (3rd Ed.)	MM
"	The Medical, Surgical, and Hygienic Treatment of Disease of Women, Especially Those Causing Sterility. [2nd Ed.]	TH
"	The Medical, Surgical, and Hygienic Treatment of Disease of Women, Especially Those Causing Sterility. [2nd Ed.]	MM
"	Materia Medica and Special Therapeutics of the New Remedies Vol.1	MM

"	Materia Medica and Special Therapeutics of the New Remedies Vol. 2	
Hansel J.	Ephedra sinensis	
Hansen O.	A Text-Book of Materia Medica and Therapeutics of Rare Remedies: A Supplement to A. G. Cowperthwaite's "Materia Medica"	MM
Harndall J. S.	Homeopathy in Veterinary Practice	PH
Hart	Therapeutics of Nervous Diseases	TH
Hawkes William J.	Characteristic Indications for Prominent Remedies	MM
Heal Thyself	1933-1940	JO
Helmuth William Tod	Surgery and its Adaptation to Homeopathic Practice	TH
Hempel Charles Julius	A New and Comprehensive System of Materia Medica Vol 1 & Vol 2	CL
Hering C.	Guiding Symptoms of our Materia Medica (10 vols.)	MM
Hering C.	The Homeopathic Domestic Physician	TH
Hering C. & Martin H. N.	The Journal of Homeopathic Clinics (Vol 1 and 2)	

Herrick Nancy	Animal Mind, Human Voices: Proving of Eight New Animal Remedies	PR
Herscu P.	The Homeopathic Treatment of Children Stramonium	
"		
Hill B. L. and Hunt Jas. G.	The Homeopathic Practice of Surgery, Together with Operative Surgery	TH
Hind J.	Chronic Diseases and Theory of Miasms	TH
The Homeopathic Herald	1940-1955	JO
The Homeopathic Medical Society	1888	JO
Homeopathic Medical Society of the State of New York, Transactions	1911 Volume LV	JO
	1913 Volume LVII	JO
	1915 Volume LIX	JO
	1916 Volume LX	JO
Homeopathic Record	11/1858 – 1859	JO

The Homeopathic World	1931 – 1932	JO
Homeopathic World	1915 Volume V – Number 1	JO
Homeopathician (A Journal for Pure Homeopathy)	1914 Volume IV – Number 1 to 2	JO
Homeopathician (A Journal for Pure Homeopathy)	138	JO
Homeopathy		JO
Homeopathic LINKS	1994-1999	JO
The Homeopathic Recorder	1910 Vol. XXV (Numbers 1 to 12)	JO
,,	1911 Vol. XXVI (Numbers 1 to 12)	JO
,,	1912 Vol. XXVII (Numbers 1 to 12)	JO
,,	1913, 1918, 1920, 1923	JO
,,	1925 Volume XL, December	JO
,,	1926-1927	JO
,,	1930-1932	JO
,,	1935-1936	JO

	1939-1940	JO
	1943-1945	JO
	1948-1955	JO

Houghton Jacqueline and Halahan Elisabeth	The Homeopathic Proving of Lac humanum	RE
		PR
Hoyne T. S.	MM Clinical Therapeutics (2 vols.)	
Hughes Richard	A Manual of Therapeutics: According to the Method of Hahnemann	CL
"	The Principles and Practice of Homeopathy	PH
"	Manual of Pharamacodynamics	MM
Hughes R. and Dake J. P.	A Cyclopedia of Drug Pathogenesy 4 Vols.	MM
Hutchison J. W.	700 Redline Symptoms	MM
Indian Journal of Homeopathic Medicine	1995-1996	JO
International Foundation for Homeopathy: Case Conference Proceedings	1990-1995	JO

International Hahnemannian Association	1907 1911-1913	JO
International Homeopathic Research Trust	1948	JO
Jahr G. H. G.	Homeopathic Treatment of the Diseases of Females and Infants at the Breast	TH
,,	Venereal Diseases, their Pathological Nature, Correct Diagnosis and Homeopathic Treatment	TH
,,	40 Years of Homeopathic Practice	TH
Jollyman N. W.	Asthma: Causes, Types & Homeopathic Treatment	TH
Jones Eli G.	Cancer (Its Causes, Symptoms & Treatment)	TH
Julian O. A.	Materia Medica of Nosodes	
Julian O. A.	Materia Medica of New Homeopathic Remedies	MM
Kamthan P. S.	The Hemorrhage Controller	TH
,,	The Female Prescriber	TH
,,	Specific Remedies for Respiratory, Cardiac and Urinary Diseases	TH

,,	Remedies for Skin and Bones Diseases	TH
Kamthan P. S.	Remedies for Pain and Warts	TH
,,	How to Cure Headache, Facial Neuralgia, Glaucoma, Toothache	TH
,,		TH
,,	How Homeopathy Cures Mania, Melancholia and Madness	TH
,,	Gout, Arthiritis and Rheumatism with Concomitants	TH
,,	CANCER – Curable under Homeopathic Treatment	
Kamthan S. K.	First Aid Prescriber	TH
Kansal Kamal	The Biochemic Remedies	TH
,,	Homeopathic Treatement - Pet Animals	TH
,,	Diabetes Mellitus	TH
,,	Dental Diseases	TH
,,	Constipation	TH
Kent James Tyler	New Remedies, Clinical Cases, Lesser Writings, Aphorisms and Precepts	CL
,,		PH
,,	Use of the Repertory "How to Study the Repertory"	PH

,,	What the Doctor Needs of Know in Order to Make a Successful Prescription	
,,	Lectures from Dunham College	MM
,,	Lectures on Homeopathic Materia Medica Kent's Lectures on Homeopathic Philosophy	PH
Klein Louis	Loxosceles Reclusa – The Brown Recluse Spider	PR
,,	Helodrilus caliginosus – Information and Synopsis of a New Proving	PR
Klein Louis	Carbon Dioxide	PR
,,	Coriandrum Proving	PR
Klein Louis and Mantewsiwich Emily	Hahnemanian Proving of Argentum Sulphuricum	PR
Knerr C. B.	Drugs Relationships	MM
Krishna Kumar P.	The Woman, Female Problems and their Cure	MM
,,	The Man, Sexual Problems and their Cure	MM
,,	Talks on Poisons, Metals Acids & Nosodes Used as Homeopathic Medicines	MM

Krishnamooty V. K.	Homeopathy Accidents Injuries	TH
Kulkarni V.	Gynecology and Obstetrics Therapeutics	TH
Laurie Joseph	An Epitome of the Homeopathic Domestic Medicine. Enlarged and Improved by A. Gerard Hull.	TH
"	The Homeopathic Domestic Medicine Vol 1 & Vol 2	CL
Leeser Otto	Text Book of Materia Medica	MM
Le Roux Patricia	The Acids	PR
Le Roux Patricia	Lac Caninum, Remedy of Ailments from Child Sexual Abuse.	MM
Liga Medicorum Homeopathica Internationlis	24th Congress - Hamburg - 1979	JO
"	43rd Congress - Athens - 1988	JO
"	45th Congress - Barcelona - 1990	JO
Lilienthal Samuel	Homeopathic Therapeutics	TH
Lippe A. von	Keynotes of the Homeopathic Materia Medica	MM

"	Keynotes & Redline Symptoms of Materia Medica	MM
Lippe C.	Textbook of Materia Medica	MM
Lustig Didier and Rey Jacques	The Proving of Neptunium muriarticum	PR
Macfarlan Donald	Concise Pictures of Dynamised Drugs Personally Proven	MM
Majumdar P. C.	Appendicitis Curable by Medicine	TH
Malhotra H. C.	Menses and Health (A Lady's Manual of Homeopathic Care)	TH
"	Fistula, Piles - Care and Treatment	TH
Marim Matheus	Simplified Materia Medica of Bothrops jararacussu	CL
Master Farokh Jamshed	Homeopathic Treatment of Acute Cardio-Respiratory Failure	TH
"	Tumours and Homeopathy	PH
"	Tubercular Miasm Tuberculins	MM
"	The Web Spinners	
"	The State of Mind that Affects Fetus	TH
"	The Fascinating Fungi	MM

,,	The Bed Side Organon of Medicine	PH
,,	Diseases of the Skin (Including of Exanthemata)	
,,	Sycotic Shame	
Master Farokh Jamshed	Suppressed Staphysagria	MM
,,	S. Ignatius Bean	MM
,,	Snakes in Homeopathic Grass	MM
,,	Sandy Silicea	MM
,,	Perceiving Rubrics of the Mind	RE
,,	Naja Naja Naja	MM
,,	Mysterious Thuja	MM
,,	Lycopodium	MM
,,	Homeopathy in Cervical Spondylosis	
,,	Homeopathy in Cancer	TH
,,	Homeopathic Dictionary of Dreams	TH
,,	Hair Loss	TH
,,	Bed-Wetting (Enuresis)	TH

"	Ammonium the Sour Prunes	MM
"	Agitated Argentums	
"	A Proving of Moccasin Snake Toxicophis)	MM
Mathur K. N.	Diabetes Mellitus Its Diagnosis & Treatment	TH
"	Systematic Materia Medica of Homeopathic Remedies	MM
Mathur R. P.	Common Infectious Diseases with Therapeutic & Repertory in Homeopathy	TH
Medical Advance 1887 Vol XIX (7-12)		JO
"	1888 Vol XX - Part 1 (1-7)	JO
"	1889 Volume XXII (1-6) Volume XXIII (7-12)	JO
Moffat J. L.	Homeopathic Therapeutics in Ophthalmology	TH
Mohanty Niranjan	Text Book of Homeopathic Materia Medica	MM
Moore James	Dog Diseases Treated by Homeopathy	TH
Morgan William	The Signs and Concomitant Derangements of Pregnancy	TH

"	Diphteria (Its History, Causes, Symptoms, Diagnosis, Pathology and Treatment)	TH
"	Homeopathic Treatment of Indigestion, Constipation, and Hemorrhoids	TH
"	Diabetes Mellitus	TH
Morrison R.	Seminar Burgh Haamstede Sept 1987	CA
"	Desktop Companion to Physical Pathology	TH
"	Burgh-Haamstede 1988 (Seminar Part 2)	CA
Morrison R. and Nancy Herrick	Netherlands November 1991	CA
Mount S. J. L.	Migraine	TH
Müller Karl-Josef	Argentum nitricum Cases	CL
"	Carcinosinum	CL
"	Lac caninum	CL
"	Lac felinum Cases	CL
"	Moschus cases Opimum Cases	CL
"	Phosphoric Acid Cases	CL

Müller Karl-Josef	Tegenaria artica Cases	CL
"	The Female Lycopodium	CL
Müller Karl-Josef	Thuja Occidentalis [New Aspects of the Remedy with Clinical Information]	CL
"	Tyrannosaurus rex Cases	CL
Murphy R.	Homeopathic Remedy Guide (Lotus Materia Medica)	MM
"	Extractions of "Homeopathic Medical Repertory"	EX
Narasimhamruti	Handbook of Materia Medica and Therapeutics of Homeopathy	
Nash E. B.	Leaders in Respiratory Organs	TH
"	Leaders in Typhoid Fever	TH
"	Leaders for the Use of Sulphur with Comparisons	MM
"	Nash Expanded Work	MM
"	Regional Leaders	MM
"	Testimony of the Clinic	MM
Neesgard Per	Hypothesis Collection - Primary Psora and Miasmatic Dynamic	

Neustaedter Randall	Clematis Proving	PR
New England Journal of Homeopathy	Volume 5, Number 4 1998	JO
Norland Misha	Collected Provings	PR
North American Journal of Homeopathy	1923	JO
Norton A. B.	Ophthalmic Diseases and Therapeutics	CL
O' Connor Joseph T.	The American Homeopathic Pharmacopoeia [2nd Ed.]	MM
Olsen Steve	Trees and Plants that Heal	PR
The Organon	1878-1881	JO
Ortega P.S.	Notes on Miasms	PH
Ostrom Homer Irvin	Leucorrhea and other Varieties of Gynaecological Catarrh	TH
Pacific Coast Journal of Homeopathy	1917 (April to December) Numbers 4 to 12	JO
"	1937	JO
Paige W. H.	Diseases of the Lungs Bronchi & Pleura	TH

Palsule S. G.	Homeopathic Treatment for E.N.T. Diseases	TH
,,	Dentistry and Homeopathy	TH
,,	Asthma and Blood Pressure	TH
Panda B. B.	Significance of Dreams in Homeopathic Prescribing	TH
Paterson J.	The Bowels Nosodes	XX
Paul	Skin	MM
Pavri Keki R. S.	Essentials of Diabetes Mellitus	MM
Peters John C.	A Complete Treatise on Headaches and Diseases of the Head	CL
Peters John C.	A Treatise on the Inflammatory and Organic Diseases of the Brain	CL
Petersen Fred Julius	Materia Medica and Clinical Therapeutics	CL
Phatak S. R.	Materia Medica of Homeopathic Medicines	MM
Poirier Jean	Homeopathic Treatment of the Diseases of Heart	TH
Pulford A.	Homeopathic Materia Medica of Graphic Drug, Pictures and Clinical Comments	TH

"	Homeopathic Leaders in Pneumonia	TH
Quinquennial Homeopathic International Congress, Transactions of the Eighth	(Vol 1) 1911	JO
" Ninth	1927	JO
Radar Keynotes	Radar Keynotes Version 4 - Characteristics and Pecularities - A Compiled Materia Medica	KN
Rajagopalarao P.	Most Valuable Tips from Masters of Homeopathy	TH
Ramseyer A. A.	Rademacher's Universal & Organ Remedies	MM
Rastogi	Homeopathic Gems Materia Medica	MM
Rastogi D.P.	Use of Indigenous and Other Remedies in Homeopathy as Home Remedies	TH
Rastogi D. P.	Some Case Reports	CA
Raue C. G.	Diseases of Children	TH
Rawat P. S.	Homeopathy in Angina Pectoris	TH
Rawat P. S.	Homeopathy in Acne & Alopecia	TH

Richardson-Boedler	The Psychological / Constitutional Essences of the Bach Flower Remedies	MM
"	Bach Flower Remedies - Catalysts in Homeopathic Cure	TH
Riley D.	Provings	
Rísquez F.	Psychiatry and Homeopathy	PH
Roberts H. A.	The Study of Remedies by Comparison	MM
"	The Rheumatic Remedies	MM
"	Sensation As If	TH
"	The Principles and Art of Cure by Homeopathy - A Modern Textbook	PH
"	The Spider Poisons	MM
Roberts H. A. and Wilson A. C.	The Principles and Practicability of Boenninghausen's Therapeutic Pocket Book	PH
Rollin R. Gregg	An Illustrated Repertory of Pains in Chest, Sides and Back: Their Direction and Character, Confirmed by Clinical Cases. [2nd Ed.]	RE
Rossertti Luiz	Lepidoptera saturniidae	PR
Rowe Todd	A Proving of Argemone pleicantha	PR

"	Cathartes aura: A Proving of Turkey Vulture	PR
"	Urolophus halleri (A Proving of Round Stingray)	PR
"	Heloderma Suspectum	PR
Rowe Todd	Carnegia Gibantea (A Proving of Saguaro Cactus)	PR
Royal G.	The Textbook of Homeopathic Materia Medica	MM
Ruddock E. H.	The Pocket Manual of Homeopathic Veterinary Medicine	TH
"	The Common Diseases of Women	TH
Ruddock E. H.	The Common Diseases of Children	TH
"	Homeopathic Treatment of Infants and Children	TH
Rush John	The Handbook of Veterinary Homeopathy	
Saine A.	Psychiatric Patients (Hahnemann and Psychological Cases, Lectures on Pure Classical Homeopathy)	
Samuel	Keynotes	MM
Sankaran Rajan	The Substance of Homeopathy	PH

"	The Spirit of Homeopathy	
"	The Soul of Remedies	MM
"	Provings	PR
Santwani M. T.	Common Ailments of Children and Their Homeopathic Management	TH
Satya Paul	Analogy of Pain	Cl re
Savulescu Geo and Crump Sue	Proving Quercus Robur	PR
Schadde Anne	Proving of Ozone	PR
Schmidt P.	The Hidden Treasures of the Last Organon	PH
"	The Art of Interrogation	PH
"	The Art of Case Taking	PH
"	Defective Illness	TH
Scholten J.	Homeopathy and the Elements	MM
"	Homeopathy and Minerals	MM
Schulz Elisabeth	Buteo jamaicensis - Hawk	PR
"	Columba palumbus	PR

"	Cygnus olor	PR
Schultz Elisabeth	Falco cherrug	PR
"	Test Flight	PR
"	Vultur gryphus - Condor	PR
Schwartz W. H.	Homeopathic Medical Treatment of Wounds and Injuries	
Shah Ronak J.	Veratrum - An Egoistic Lily [1st Ed.]	CL
Sherr Jeremy	The Dynamic and Methodology of Homeopathic Provings	PH
"	The Homeopathic Proving of Plutonium nitricum, Including the Toxicology of Ionising Radiation	PR
"	Dynamic Provings Volume 1	PR
"	Proving of Hydrogen	PR
"	The Homeopathic Proving of Scorpio	PR
Shore J.	Seminar Scotland 1989	CA
"	Seminar Hapert September 1990	CA
"	Seminar Hapert April 1991	CA
"	Seminar Glasgow April 1990	

Shreedharan C. K	A Concise Materia Medica & Repertory of Nosodes	MM
Singh Sapuran	Hering's Model Cures	
Sivaraman M. S.	Homeopathic Treatment of Asthma	TH
Sivaraman P.	Hemorrhoids Cured by Homeopathic Medicines	MM
"	Epilepsy Cured with Homeopathic Medicines	MM
"	Ear, Nose and Throat	MM
"	Dreams and their Homeopathic Medicines	TH
"	Asthma Cured with Homeop. Medicines	MM
Skinner T.	Homeopathy in its Relation to the Diseases of Females or Gynaecology	TH
Small A.E.	Manual of Homeopathic Practice, for the Use of Families and Private Individuals [9th Ed. Enlarged]	TH
Snowdon Janet	Dreaming Potency	PR
Sonz Susan and Stewart Robet	The Proving of Musca domestica	PR
Souk-Aloun Phou	Unintentional Provings	PR

"	Provings of the French "Comitéd" Expérimentation Homéopathique"	PR
Stephenson J.	Hahnemannian Provings Hyganthropharmacology (A materia Medica and Repertory)	MM
Stirling Penelope	The Homeopathic Provin of Crack Willow: Salix Fragilis	PR
Sudarshan S. R.	Homeopathic Treatment of Non-Malarial Fevers	MM
Sukumaran N.	Heart Problems of Adults and Aged	TH
Swan Samuel	Proving Of Ovi Gallina Pellicula-Membrane Of The Egg Shell	PR
Swayanadan K. R.	Intestinal Worms	MM
Synthesis 7.0	Extractions	EX
Teste A.	The Homeopathic Materia Medica	MM
Tiwari Shashi Kant	Homeopathy and Child Care: Principles, Therapeutics, Children's Type, Repertory	RE
TH Tws 1 Twohig Julia	"Deadly Romance" A homeopathic Proving Latrodectus hasseltii-Red Back Spider	PR
Tyler Margaret	Different Ways of Findings the Remedy	PH

"	Hahnemann's Conception of Chronic Disease, as Caused by Parasitic Micro-Organisms	CL
"		PH
"	Repertorizing	TH
"	Pointers to the Common Remedies	MM
"	Drosera	MM
Vakil P.	Acute Conditions, Injuries, etc.	TH
Varma P. N. and Indu Vaid	A Text Book of Homeopathic Therapeutics: Vol 1: Therapeutics of the Central Nervous System	
"	Encyclopedia of Homeopathic Pharmacopoeia - 2 Vols.	TH
Vermeulen Frans	Side Effects	MM
"	Synoptic Materia Medica 1	MM
"	Synoptic Materia Medica 2	MM
"	Concordant Materia Medica	MM
"	Prisma - The Arcana of Materia Medica Illuminated - Similars and Parallels Between Substance and Remedy	
Vithoulkas George	The Essence of Materia Medica	MM

"	Talks on Classical Homeopathy - The Esalen Conferences 1980 Part I, II & III	TH
"	Materia Medica Viva (7 Vols.)	MM
Vithoulkas George and Olsen Steve	Winning Strategies of Case Analysis: A Short Course For Radar and the Vithoulkas Expert System	PH
Wadia S. R.	Tonsilitis Cured by Homeopathy	TH
Wadia S. R.	Leucoderma (Its Homeopathic Treatment)	TH
"	Homeopathy in Children's Diseases	TH
"	Homeopathy Cures Asthma	TH
Ward J. W.	Unabridged Dictionary of the Sensation "As If" Vol 1	TH
"	Unabridged Dictionary of the Sensation "As If" Vol 2	TH
Wheeler C. E.	Introduction to the Principles of Homeopathy	MM
Wilkinson Chris	Hekla Lava	PR
"	The Homeopathic Proving of Alabaster	PR

"	The Homeopathic Proving of Venus Stella Errans	PR
Woods F. H.	Essentials of Homeopathic Prscribing	MM
Woodward A. W.	Constitutional Therapeutics	TH
World Congress of Homeopathic Physicians and Surgeons, Transactions of	1893	JO
Wright Craig	Bitis arietans and its Venum (Clotho arietans)	PR
Wright Elisabeth	A Brief Study Course in Homeopathy	PH
Yasgur Jay	Homeopathic Dictionary	
Yingling W. A.	The Accouchers Emergency Manual	MM
Zaren A.	Seminar Lelystad, May 1989	CA

APPENDIX - B

BOOKS IN REFERENCE WORKS LIBRARY

PROVINGS:

Allen, H. C: Materia Medica with the Nosodes and X-Ray
Allen, TF: Encyclopedia of Pure Materia Medica (10)
Anshutz, EP: New, Old and Forgotten Remedies
Azar & Marlow-Fries: Ruby Proving
Bedayn, G: Corvus Corax Principalis (Raven) Proving
Birch, K and Rockwell J: Sequoia Sempervirens (Redwood) Proving
Black, G: Viscum Album (Miostletoe) Proving
Bond, A: Tungsten Proving
Bradford, TL: Index to Homeopathic Provings
Central Council for Research in Homeopathy: Aegle Folia Proving
Central Council for Research in Homeopathy: Aegle Marmelos Proving
Collier, C. & Davis, J: Lavendula Vera Proving
Deacon & Ribot-Smith: Spagyrical Proving of Bellis Perennis
Dransfield, G: Spectrum Proving
Eising, N: Ignis Alcoholics & Succinum (Fire & Amber) Provings
Eising, N: Granite Proving
Eising, N: Limestone Proving
Eising, N: Marble Proving
Ghose, SC: Drugs of Hindustan
Gray, A: Chironex Fleckeri (Box Jellyfish) Proving
Gray, A: Moreton Bay Fig Proving

Grimes, M: Galeocerdo Cuvier Hepar (Tiger Shark Liver) Proving
Guild of Homeopaths: Meditation Provings from Prometheus
Hahnemann, S: Materia Medica Pura
Hahnemann, SC: Chronic Diseases
Hale, EM: Saw Palmetto and Therapeutic Applications
Hammond, D: MDMA Proving
Helios: Hadrian's Wall Proving
Herrick, N: Animal Minds Human Voices
Herrick, N: Lac Delphinum Proving
Herrick, N: Lac Equinum Proving
Houghton & Halahan: Proving of Lac Humanum
Hughes Medical Club: Gelsemium
Irwin, A: Seven Streams of Taosca Proving
Julian, OA : Materia Medica of New Homeopathic Remedies
King, L and Lawrence, B: Luna Proving
Klein, L: Argentum Sulphuricum Proving
Klein, Loxosceles Reclusa (Brown Recluse) Proving
Klein, L: Carbon Dioxide
Proving Klein, L: Coriandrum (Coriander)
Proving Klein, L: Helodrilus (Earthworm) Proving
Koenig & Santos : Berberis, Rhododendron, Convallaria Provings
Marcy, Peters & Fullgraff: New Provings & Clinical Experiences
Macfarlane, D: Dynamised Drugs
Macfarlane, D: Provings
Mc Clintock, L: Lac Glama (Llama Milk) Proving
Medical Investigation Club of Baltimore: Pathogenic MM
Metcalf, JW: Homeopathic Provings
Mure, B: Animal and Vegetable Poisons of the Brazilian Empire
Neustaedter, R: Clematis Proving
New York School of Homeopathy: Musca Domestica (Fly) Proving
Olsen, S: Trees and Plants That Heal

Palmer, S: Aqua Tunbridge Wells Proving
Riley, D: New Provings
Rimmler, U: Vulture Gryphus (Condor) Proving
Robbins, P: Phascolarctos Cinereus (Koala) Proving
Robertson, F: Mandragora Proving
Rowe, T: Carnegia Gigantea (Saguaro Cactus) Proving
Rowe, T: Catharthes Aura (Turkey Vulture) Proving
Rowe, T: Heloderma Suspectum (Gila Monster) Proving
Rowe, T: Urolophus Halleri (Stingray) Proving
South Downs School of Homeopathy: Chlamydia Proving
South Downs School of Homeopathy: Mobile Phone Radiation Proving
Sankaran, R: Provings
Schadde, A: Cypraea Eglantina (Cowrie Snail) Proving
Schadde, A: Ginkgo Biloba Proving
Schadde, A: Lapis Lazuli Proving
Schadde, A: Ozone Proving
School of Homeopathy: Agathis Australis (Kauri tree) Proving
School of Homeopathy: AIDS Proving
School of Homeopathy: Falco Peregrinus Disciplinatus (Falcon) Proving
School of Homeopathy: LSD Proving
School of Homeopathy: N. Wales Slate Proving
School of Homeopathy: Oak Galls Proving
School of Homeopathy: Positronium (Antimatter) Proving
School of Homeopathy: Salix Fragilis (Crack Willow) Proving
School of Homeopathy: Sunset Lava
School of Homeopathy: Ubulawo Proving
Schuster, B: Bambusa Arundinacea (Bamboo) Proving
Schuster, B: Cola Nitida (Kola Nut) Proving
Schultz, E: Vultur Gryphus (Condor) Proving

Schultz, E: Falco Cherrug (Falcon) Proving
Schultz, E: Holy Ibis Proving
Schultz, E: Lac Humanum Proving I
Schultz, E: Lac Humanum Proving II
Schultz, E: Radium Bromatum Proving
Schultz, E: Buteo Jamaicensis (Redtail Hawk) Proving
Schultz, E: Columba Palumbus (Ring-Dove) Proving
Schultz, E: Cygnus Olor (Swan) Proving
Scriven, D and Daws, J: Sol Proving
Shah, J: Rattus Rattus (Rat) Proving
Sherr, J: Chocolate Proving
Sherr, J: Dynamic Provings I
Sherr, J: Hydrogen Proving
Shore, J: Atrax Robustus (Australian mygale spider) Proving
Shore, J: Buteo Jamaicensis (Rdtail Hawk) Proving
Shore, J: Columba Palumbus (Ring-necked Dove) Proving
Shore, J: Haliaeetus Leucocephalus (Bald Eagle) Proving
Shore, J: Scarlet Macaw Proving
Souk-Aloun, P: Pathogenesis of Brucella Melitensis and Melitococcinum Proving
Souk-Aloun, P: Propranolol Proving
Souk-Aloun, P: Unintentional Provings
Sowton, C: Tela Aranea (Spiderweb) Proving
Stephenson, J: Hahnemannian Provings
Sujit, C: Ficus Indica (Banyan) Proving
Sujit, C: Chocolate Proving
Sunil, A and Shah, N: Benzinum Petroleum Proving
Swan, S: A Materia Medica Containing Provings and Clinical Verifications of Nosodes and Morbific Products
Tumminello, PL: Rhus Glabra Proving
Vakil, P: Leprominum Proving

Wichman, J: Fagus Sylvatica Proving
Wilkinson: Alabaster Proving

CLINICAL CASES:

Burnett, JC: Fifty Reasons for Being a Homeopath
Case, EE : Some Clinical Experiences of E.E. Case with Selected Writings
Chipkin, P: Clinical Cases
Contemporary Clinic Cases
Fleisher, M: Clinical Cases
Ghosh, SK: Clinical Experience With Some Rare Nosodes
Gray, B: Clinical Cases
Heron, K: Clinical Cases
Herrick, N: Clinical Cases
International Foundation for Homeopathy Proceedings: 1991
International Foundation for Homeopathy Proceedings: 1992
International Foundation for Homeopathy Proceedings: 1993
International Foundation for Homeopathy Proceedings: 1994
International Foundation for Homeopathy Proceedings: 1995
Italiano, M: Cured Cases
Johnston, L: Clinical Cases
Kent, JT: Clinical Cases
Koenig P & S : Clinical Cases
Mangialavori, M: Clinical Cases
Morrison, R: Clinical Cases
Moskowitz, R: Resonance
Mueller, K: Apium Cases
Mueller, Argentum nitricum Cases
Mueller, K: Carcinosin Cases
Mueller, K: Laccaninum Cases
Mueller, K: Lac felinum Cases

Mueller, K: Moschus Cases
Mueller, K: Phosphoric Acid Cases
Mueller, K: Tegenaria atrica Cases
Mueller, K: Thuja Cases
Mueller, K: Tyrannosaurus rex Cases
Nash, EB: Testimony of the Clinic
Owen, J: Clinical Cases
Rastogi, DP: Case Reports
Reichenberg-Ullman, J: Clinical Cases
Shore, J: Clinical Cases
Singh, S: Hering's Model Cures
Tessler: Scutellaria Cases
Thompson, M: Cases & Misc.
Ullman, B: Clinical Cases
Ullman, B & Reichenberg-Ullman, J: Prozac Free Cases
Warkentin, L: Animal Cases

CHARACTERISTIC MATERIA MEDICA:

Allen, HC : Keynotes to the Materia Medica
Allen, TF: A Primer of Materia Medica for Practitioner of Homeopathy
Boenninghausen, CMF Von: Characteristics
Boericke, W: Pocket Manual of Homeopathic Materia Medica
Boger, CM: Synoptic Key of The Materia Medica
Breyfogle, WL : Epitome of Homeopathic Medicines
Buck, H: Outlines of Materia Medica
Choudhuri, NM : A Study on Materia Medica
Cleveland, CL: Salient Materia Medica
Douglass, ME : Pearls of Homeopathy
Farrington, EA : Therapeutic Pointers
Guernsey, HN : Key-Notes to the Materia Medica

Guess, G: KHA Confirmatories
Hawkes, WJ MD : Characteristic Indications for 100 Remedies
Hering, C: Condensed Materia Medica
Le Roux, P: Acids
Lippe, A: Key Notes and Red Line Symptoms of the Materia Medica
Mangialavori, M: Repertory Additions
Morrison, R: Desktop Guide To Keynotes & Confirmatory Symptoms
Murphy, R: Homeopathic Remedy Guide (formerly Lotus Materia Medica)
Niederkorn, JS: A Handy Reference Book
Phatak, SR: Materia Medica of Homeopathic Remedies
Pulford, A: Key To The Homeopathic Materia Medica
Ramiah, NK: Forty Tissue Remedies
Rastogi, DP: Homeopathic Gems
Skinner, T: Grand Characteristics of The Materia Medica
Tyler, ML: Homeopathic Drug Pictures
Vermeulen, F: Synoptic Materia Medica I
Vermeulen, F: Synoptic Materia Medica II
Wood, JC : Essentials of Homeopathic Prescribring

GENERAL MATERIA MEDICA:

Allen, TF : Hand Book of MM And Homeopathic Therapeutics
Arndt, HR: First Lessons in the Symptomatology of Leading Homeopathic Remedies
Bechet & Espanet : Manual of Homeopathy
Blackie, M: Comparison of Ars, Nit-ac, Hepar and Nux
Blackwood, AL : A Manual of Materia Medica, Therapeutics and Pharmacology
Brefogle, W. : Epitome of Homeopathic Medicines
Burnett, JC: Gold in Organic Heart Disease

Burnett, JC: Natrum Muriaticum as Test of the Doctrine of Drug Dynamization
Burnett, JC: On Vaccinosis and Its Cure by Thuja Occidentalis
Burt, WH: Characteristic Materia Medica
Burt, WH: Physiological Materia Medica
Clark, GH: ABC Manual of Materia Medica and Therapeutics
Clarke, AG: Decachords
Clarke, JH: Constitutional Medicine
Clarke, JH: Dictionary of Practical Materia Medica (3)
Clarke, JH: Gunpower as a War Remedy
Clarke, JH : Hemorrhoids and Habitual Constipation
Clarke, JC: Therapeutics of the Serpent Poisons
Clarke, JH: Radium as an Internal Remedy
Cowperthwaite, AC: Textbook of Materia Medica and Therapeutics
Crandall, OH: Diseases and their Cure by Homeopathy and Biochemistry: Fifty Years' Experience
Curie, PF: Practice of Homeopathy
Desai, R: Magnificant Plants 1
Desai, R: Magnificant Plants 2
Dewey, WA: Essentials of Homeopathic Materia Medica and Homeopathic Pharmacy
Dewey, WA : Practical Homeopathic Therapeutics
Digby, BW: Homeopathic Lectures
Douglass, ME : Characteristics of the Homeopathic Materia Medica
Dunham, C: The Science of Therapeutics
Enz, EE: Pathogenetic Materia Medica
Fahnestock, JC: A Manual of Homeopathic MM
Farrington, EA : Supplement To Gross' Comparative Materia Medica
Farrington, EA: Homeopathy and Homeopathic Prescribing
Farrington, EA: Lesser Writings with Therapeutic Hints

Foubister, DM: The Carcinosin Drug Picture
Foubister, DM: Therapeutic Hints for Students of Homeopathy
Fyfe, JW: The Essentials Of Modern Materia Medica And Therapeutics
Gallavardin, JP: Psychic Medicines
Gibson, DM: Studies of Homeopathic Remedies
Gladwin, FE: People of the Materia Medica World
Gross, RH: Comparative Materia Medica
Grimmer, AH: The Collected Works of Arthur Hill Grimmer, MD
Guernsey, HN: Lectures on the Materia Medica
Gunavante: The Genius of Homeopathic Remedies
Gutman, W: Homeopathy, the Fundamentals of Its Philosophy, the Essence of Its Remedies
Hahnemann, SC: Treatise on the Effects of Coffee
Hale, EM: Materia Medica & Special Therapeutics of the New Remedies 1
Hale, EM: Materia Medica & Special Therapeutics of the New Remedies 2
Hanchett, HG: Elements of Modern Domestic Medicine
Hansen, O: Textbook of Rate Homeopathic Remedies
Hartmann, F: Practical Observations on Some of the Chief Homeopathic Remedies
Hawkes, WJ: Characteristic Indications for Prominent Remedies
Heinigke, C: Pathogenetic Outline of Homeopathic Drugs
Hempel, CG: A New and Comprehensive System of Materia Medica and Therapeutics
Hering, C: Guiding Symptoms of Our Materia Medica (10)
Hubbard, EW: Articles
Hughes, R & Dake, J: Cyclopedia of Drug Pathogensy (3)
Hughes, R: A Manual of Pharmacodynamics
Hughes, R: The Knowledge of the Physician: Lectures

Hutchison, JW : Seven Hundred Red Line Symptoms of Cowperthwaite
Jahr, GHG: New Manual of Homeopathic Practice
Johnson, ID: Therapeutic Key, or Practical Guide for the Treatment of Acute Disease
Jones, S : The Medical Genius
Julian, OA: Intestinal Nosodes of Bach - Paterson
Julian, OA: Materia Medica of the Nosodes
Kent, JT : Lectures On Homeopathic Materia Medica
Laurie, J : The Homeopathic Practice of Medicine
Lesser, O: Textbook of Inorganic Medicinal Substances
Lilienthal, S: Homeopathic Therapeutics
Lippe, A: Keynotes of the Homeopathic Materia Medica
Lippe, A: Textbook of Materia Medica
Luyties Characteristic Materia Medica and Condensed Clinical Index (compilation)
Marsh, A: Clinical Drug Pictures
Master, F: Agitated Argentums
Master, F: Fascinating Fungi
Master, F: Mysterious Thuja
Master, F: Naja
Master, F: Sycotic Shame
Master, F: Web Spinners
Mathur, KN: Systematic Materia Medica of Homeopathic Remedies
Mirilli, J: Thematic Repertory and Materia Medica of the Mind Symptoms
Monroe, AL: Materia Medica Memorizer
Nash, EB: Leaders for the Use of Sulphur with Comparisons
Nash, EB: Leader in Homeopathic Therapeutics

Nash, EB: Radium
Nash, EB: Regional Leaders
Patersimilias: A Song of Symptoms
Paterson, J: Bowel Nosodes
Petersen, O: Therapeutics Pharmacopoeia
Pierce, W: Plain Talks On Materia Medica With Comparisons
Puddephatt, N & Kincaid-Smith, M: Sign Posts to the Homeopathic Remedies
Puhlmann, CG: Handbook of Homeopathic Practice
Pulford, A: Graphic Drug Pictures and Clinical Comments
Pulte, JH: Homeopathic Domestic Physician
Rastogi, DP: Use Of Indigenous And Other Remedies In Homeopathy As Home Remedies
Reckeweg, H: Homeopathia Antihomotoxica
Royal, G: Textbook of Materia Medica
Ruckert, EF: Homeopathic Therapeutics; or, Outlines of Successful Homeopathic Cures
Ruddock, EH: Homeopathic Vade Mecum
Ruddock, EH: The Stepping Stone to Homeopathy and Health
Sankaran, P: Random Notes On Some Remedies
Sankaran, P: Some Notes On the Nosodes
Sankaran, P: The Indications & Uses of the Bowel Nosodes
Sankaran, R: The Spirit of Homeopathy
Sankaran, R: The Soul of Remedies
Sankaran, R: The Substance of Homeopathy
Schmidt, P: Defective Illness
Scholten, J: Homeopathy and Minerals
Shedd, PW: Clinical Repertory and Keynotes of 50 Polychrests
Shepherd, D: A Physician's Posy
Shepherd, D: Homeopathy in Epidemic Diseases
Shepherd, D: More Magic of the Minimum Dose

Smith, AD: The Home Prescriber Domestic Guide
Snelling: Symptomatology
Speight, P: A Study Course in Homeopathy
Stapf, JE: Additions to the MM Pura
Stephenson, J: A Doctor's Guide to Helping Yourself with Homeopathic Remedies
Teste, A: The Homeopathic Materia Medica, Arranged Systematically and Practically
Thompson, M: Snake Venoms and Homeopathy
Treuherz, F: Homeopathy in the Irish Potato Famine
Tyler, ML: Drosera
Underwood, BF: MM of Differential Potency
Vermeulen, F: Concordant Materia Medica II
Weiner, M: A Comprehensive Manual of Natural Healing
Wheeler & Kenyon : Principals of Homeopathy
Whitmont, EC: Psyche & Substance
Woodbury, BC: Homeopathic Materia Medica for Nurses
Woodward, AW: Constitutional Therapeutics
Potter: New Cyclopedia of Botanical Drugs and Preparations
Yeldham, S: Homeopathy in Venereal Diseases
Mother/Child Materia Medica
Borland, DM: Children's Types
Borland, DM: Homeopathy for Mother and Infant
Burnett, JC: Change of Life in Women
Burnett, JC: Delicate, Backward, Puny and Stunted Children
Duncan, TC: Children, Acid and Alkaline
Fisher, CE: Homeopathy in Obstetric Emergencies
Foubister, DM: Homeopathy and Pediatrics
Frishmuth, J: Diseases of Childhood
Guernsey, HN: The Application of the Principles and Practice of

Homeopathy to Obstetrics and the Disorders Peculiar to Women and Young Children

Jahr, GHG: Diseases of Females, and Infants at the Breast

Leavitt, S: Homeopathic Therapeutics as Applied to Obstetrics

Minton, H: Uterine Therapeutics

Morgan, W: Pregnancy

Moskowitz, R: Homeopathic Medicines for Pregnancy & Childbirth

Ruddock, EH: The Common Diseases of Children and Their Homeopathic and General Treatment

Ruddock, EH: Lady's Manual of Homeopathic Treatment

Ruddock, EH: The Common Diseases of Women

Skinner, T: The Diseases of Females

Underwood, BF: The Diseases of Childhood with Therapeutic Indications

Van der Zee, H: Miasms in Labor

Williamson, W: Diseases of Females and Children

Wood, JC: Clinical Gynecology

Yingling, WA: Accoucheur's Emergency Manual

CLINICAL MATERIA MEDICA:

Allen, HC: Diseases and Therapeutics of the Skin

Allen, HC: Therapeutics of Intermittent Fevers

Allen, HC: Therapeutics of Tuberculous Affections

Anshutz, EP: Sexual Ills and Diseases

Bell, JB: Therapeutics of Diarrhea, Dysentry, Etc.

Berjeau, JP: Syphilis, Gonorrhea, Spermatorrhea & Urinary Diseases

Bernard, H: The Homeopathic Treatment of Constipation

Bernoville, F and Grimmer, AH: Homeopathic Treatment of Cancer
Bernard, H: The Homeopathic Treatment of of Constipation
Bernoville, F and Grimmer, AH: Homeopathic Treatment of Cancer
Bernoville, F: Remedies of the circulatory and respiratory system
Bernoville, F: Diabetes Mellitus
Bernoville, F: Eruptive Fevers and Contagious Diseases of Children
Bernoville, F: Therapeutics of the Liver and Biliary Ducts
Bernoville, F: Limits and Possibilties of Homeopathy in Biology and Mental Diseases
Bernoville, F: Chronic Rheumatism
Bernoville, F: Therapeutics of Intoxication
Blackwood, AL: Diseases of the Heart
Blackwood, AL: Diseases of the Kidneys and Nervous System
Blackwood, AL: Diseases of the Liver, Pancreas and Ductless Glands
Boenninghausen, CMF Von: Whooping Cough
Bonnerot: Ulcer of the Stomach and Duodenum
Borland, DM: Influenzas
Borland, DM: Digestive Drugs
Borland, DM: Emergencies
Borland, DM: Pneumonia
Borland, DM: Treatment of Certain Heart Conditions
Boyle, CC: Therapeutics of the Ear
Brigham, GN: Catarrhal Diseases of the Nasal/ Respiratory Organs
Buck, H: The Outlines of Regional Symptomatology
Buffum, JH: Manual of the Essentials of Diseases of the Eye and Ear

Burnett, JC: Blood Poisoning

Burnett, JC: Cataract

Burnett: JC: Consumption and Its Cure by Its Own Virus

Burnett, JC: Diseases of the Spleen

Burnett, JC: Gout and its Cure

Burnett, JC: Fistulas

Burnett, JC: The Greater Diseases of the Liver

Burnett, JC: On Neuralgia: Its Causes and Remedies

Burnett, JC: Ringworm Diseases its Constitutional Nature and Cure

Burnett, JC: Diseases of the Skin From the Organismic Standpoint

Burnett, JC: Enlarged Tonsils Cured by Medicine

Burnett, JC: Curability of Tumours

Burnett, JC: Valvular Diseases of the Heart

Burnett, JC: Organ Diseases of Women and Sterility

Burnett, JC: The Medicinal Treatment of Diseases of the Veins

Burt, WH: Therapeutics of Tuberculosis

Bushrod, WJ: Tumours

Carleton, BG: A Practical Treatise on the Disorders of the Sexual Organs of Men

Clarke, JH: The Therapeutics of Cancer

Clarke, JH: Catarrh, Colds and Grippe, Including Prevention and Cure, with Chapters on Nasal Polypus, Hay Fever and Influenza

Clarke, JH: Cholera

Clarke, JH: Diseases of the Heart and Arteries

Clarke, JH: Indigestion D Its Causes and Cure

Clarke, JH: Non-surgical Treatment of Glands and Bones

Clarke, JH: Whooping Cough

Clay, JV: Diseases of the Nose and Throat

Cooper, R: The Cancer Problem: Some Deductions based on Clinical Experience

Cowperthwaite, AC: Disorders of Menstruation

Cushing, AM: Leucorrhea, Its Concomitant Symptoms

Farrington, EA: A Clinical Materia Medica

Gallavardin, JP: Homeopathic Treatment of Alcoholism

Gentry, WD: Rubrical and Regional Text Book

Gilchrist, JG: The Homeopathic Treatment of Surgical Diseases

Grimmer, AH: Remedies That Have Cured Cancer

Guernsey, WJ: Therapeutics of Hemorrhoids

Hale, EM: Lectures On the Diseases of the Heart

Hanchett, HG: Sexual Health with Modern Homeopathic Treatment

Hart, CP: Therapeutics of Nervous Diseases

Hershoff, A: Musculoskeletal Healing

Hoyle, EP: Unneccessary Tonsil Operations

Hoyne, TS: Clinical Therapeutics

Jahr, GHG: The Venereal Diseases D Their Pathological Nature

Jessen, HC: Therapeutical Materia Medica

Kafka, J: Diseases of the Spinal Marrow and its Coverings

Karo, W: Diseases of Respiratory System

Karo, W: Diseases of the Male Genital Organs

Karo, W: Diseases of the Skin

Karo, W: Homeopathy in Women's Diseases

Karo, W: Urinary and Prostatic Troubles

Kasad, JC: Headaches and Their Concomitant Symptoms Kippax, JR: Handbook of Diseases of the Skin

Kreisberg, J: Homeopathic Handbook for Poison Ivy and Poison Oak
Lutze, FH: Facial and Sciatic Neuralgias
Moffat, JL: Homeopathic Therapeutics in Ophthalmology
Morgan, W: Diabetes Mellitus
Morgan, W: Diphtheria
Nash, EB: Leaders in Respiratory Organs
Nash EB: Leaders in Typhoid Fever
Neatby, EA: Manual of Homeopathic Therapeutics
Norton, AB: Ophthalmic Diseases and Therapeutics
Oehme, FG: Diphtheritis
Ostrom, HI : Leucorrhea and Gynaecological Catarrh
Paige, HW: Diseases of the Lungs, Bronchi and Pleura
Perkins, DC: Homeopathic Therapeutics of Rheumatism
Pierce, W: Repertory of Cough
Poirier, J: Homeopathic Treatment of the Disease of Heart
Pulford, A & DT: Monograph of Aconitum Napellus
Pulford, A & DT: Homeopathic Leaders in Pneumonia
Quay, GH: A Monograph of Diseases of the Nose and Throat
Rabe, RF: Medical Therapeutics for Daily Reference
Raue, CG: Special Pathology and Diagnostics with Therapeutic Hints
Roberts, HA: Rheumatic Remedies
Roberts, HA: The Study of Remedies by Comparison
Schwatrz, WH: The Homeopathic Medical Treatment Of Wounds And Injuries
Sharp, PH: Constipation & Diarrhea
Smith, DT : Before and After Surgical Operations

Talcott, Sh: Mental Diseases and Their Modern Treatment
Templeton, WL: Homeopathic Treatment of Influenza
Thomas, H: External Remedies
Tyler, ML & Weir, J: Remedies for Acute Conditions, Injuries, etc.
Underwood, BF: Headache
VanDenburg, MW: Therapeutics of the Respiratory System
Wells & Boenninghausen: Intermittent Fever
Wells, PP: Treatment of Diarrhea and Dysentery

REPERTORY EXTRACTIONS:

Allen, TF: Index To the Encyclopedia
Boenninghausen, CMF Von: Repertory
Boericke, O: Repertory
Clarke, JH: Clinical Repertory
Douglass, ME: Skin Diseases (Wart Section)
Knerr, CB: Repertory of Hering's Guiding Symptoms
Roberts, HA: Sensations As If
Ward, JW: Unabridged Dictionary of Sensations As If
Zandvoort, R:

JOURNALS:

American Homeopath 1995 : (14 Articles)
American Homeopath 1997 : (8 Articles)
American Homeopath 1998 : (3 Articles)
American Homeopath 1999
American Homeopath 2000
American Homeopath 2001
American Homeopath Review 1859 : (14 Articles)

American Homeopath Review 1860 : (8 Articles)
American Homeopath Review 1862 : (3 Articles)
American Homeopath Review 1863 : (8 Articles)
American Homeopath Review 1864 : (4 Articles)
American Institute of Homeopathy : (13 Articles)
The American Homeopathic Pharmacopoeia
Boyd's Homeopathic Today: : (5 Articles)
British Homeopathic Review : 1907-09 : (8 Articles)
British Homeopathic Journal : (544 Articles)
Central Journal of Homeopathy: 1924 (2 Articles)
Chironian: (16 Articles)
Cleveland Medical And Surgical Reporter: (5 Articles)
Hahnemannian Advocate: 1896, 1898-99 (229 Articles)
Hahnemannian Monthly: 1865 (4 Articles)
Hahnemannian Monthly: 1866 (6 Articles)
Hahnemannian Monthly: 1867 (5 Articles)
Hahnemannian Monthly: 1868 (19 Articles)
Hahnemannian Monthly: 1869 (25 Articles)
Hahnemannian Monthly: 1870 (19 Articles)
Hahnemannian Monthly: 1871 (6 Articles)
Hahnemannian Monthly: 1889 (6 Articles)
Hahnemannian Monthly: 1890 (19 Articles)
Hahnemannian Monthly: 1891 (5 Articles)
Hahnemannian Monthly: 1892 (5 Articles)
Hahnemannian Monthly: 1893 (8 Articles)
Hahnemannian Monthly: 1894 (7 Articles)
Heal Thyself 1933: (25 Articles)

Heal Thyself 1934: (9 Articles)
Heal Thyself 1935: (2 Articles)
Heal Thyself 1936: (8 Articles)
Heal Thyself 1945: (8 Articles)
Health Through Homeopathy: 1943: (17 Articles)
Homeopathic Links 1991: (40 Articles)
Homeopathic Links 1992: (10 Articles)
Homeopathic Links 1993: (43 Articles)
Homeopathic Links 1994: (29 Articles)
Homeopathic Links 1995: (72 Articles)
Homeopathic Links 1996: (49 Articles)
Homeopathic Links 1997: (58 Articles)
Homeopathic Links 1998: (30 Articles)
Homeopathic Links 1999: (45 Articles)
Homeopathic Links 2000: (27 Articles)
Homeopathic Medical Society: 1880 (1 Articles)
Homeopathic Physician: (554 Articles)
Homeopathic Recorder Misc: (954 Articles)
Homeopathic Recorder 1889: (85 Articles)
Homeopathic Recorder 1897: (150 Articles)
Homeopathic Recorder 1898: (154 Articles)
Homeopathic Recorder 1899: (101 Articles)
Homeopathic Recorder 1900: (91 Articles)
Homeopathic Recorder 1903: (78 Articles)
Homeopathic Recorder 1904: (55 Articles)
Homeopathic Recorder 1920: (92 Articles)
Homeopathic Recorder 1921: (31 Articles)

Homeopathic World: 1883-84, 1901-14, 1917-21, 1923-25, 1927 (247 Articles)

Homeopathy 1932: (54 Articles)

Homeopathy 1933: (69 Articles)

Homeopathy 1934: (137 Articles)

Homeopathy 1935: (171 Articles)

Homeopathy 1936: (152 Articles)

Homeopathy 1937: (109 Articles)

Homeopathy 1938: (158 Articles)

Homeopathy 1939: (14 Articles)

Homeopathy 1940: (122 Articles)

Homeopathy 1941: (182 Articles)

Homeopathy 1942: (10 Articles)

Homeopathy 1952: (32 Articles)

Homeopathy 1954: (3 Articles)

Homeopathy 1955: (5 Articles)

Homeopathy 1956: (6 Articles)

Homeopathy 1958: (5 Articles)

Homeotherapy : (141 Articles)

Homeopath, Society of Homeopaths: (50 Articles)

Homeopath Examiner: (1 Article)

Homeopathician: A Journal for Pure Homeopathy (11)

Indian Homeopathic Review 1882: (6 Articles)

Indian Homeopathic Review 1895: (54 Articles)

Indian Homeopathic Review 1896: (27 Articles)

Indian Homeopathic Review 1897: (9 Articles)

Indian Homeopathic Review 1900: (2 Articles)
Indian Homeopathic Review 1905: (9 Articles)
Indian Homeopathic Review 1908: (54 Articles)
Indian Homeopathic Review 1913: (1 Article)
Indian Homeopathic Review 1914: (11 Articles)
Indian Homeopathic Review 1915: (28 Articles)
Indian Homeopathic Review 1916: (8 Articles)
Indian Homeopathic Review 1918: (5 Articles)
Indian Homeopathic Review 1920: (1 Article)
Indian Homeopathic Review 1921: (106 Articles)
Indian Homeopathic Review 1925: (2 Articles)
Indo-German Homeopathic Review 1939: (18 Articles)
International Hahnemannian Association : (92 Articles)
Journal of the British Homeopathic Society: 1903 (1)
Layman Speaks 1972: (1 Article)
Layman Speaks 1974: (4 Articles)
Medical Advance: (256 Articles)
Medical Investigator: (2 Articles)
Medical Visitor: 1892 (4 Articles)
Mid West Homeopathic News Journal: 1928 (3 Articles)
Minneapolis Homeopathic Magazine: 1898 (1 Article)
Monthly Homeopathic Review: 1870-71, 1878, 1898, 1900, 1902 (41 Articles)
New England Medical Gazette: 1906, 1908, 1914 (10)
North American Homeopathic Journal: 1851 (21 Articles)
Pacific Coast Journal of Homeopathy: 1936, 1939, 1940 (98 Articles)

Philadelphia Journal of Homeopathy: (29 Articles)

BIOCHEMIC SALTS:

Boericke, W & Dewey, WA: Twelve Tissue Remedies of Schüssler
Carey, GW: The Biochemic System of Medicine
Chapman, JB: Dr Schussler's Biochemistry
Goltz, EG: Manual and Clinical Repertory of a Complete List of Tissue Remedies
Kulkarni, VM: The Biochemic Guide with Versified Materia Medica
Schüssler, WH: Biochemic Pocket Guide
Schüssler, WH: The Biochemical Treatment of Disease

NATURAL HISTORY:

American Pharmacopoeia 1883
Francia, Franco del: Horse Behaviour & Homeopathy
Hamilton, E: Flora Homeopathica
Millspaugh, CF: American Medicinal Plants
Natural History of Animals
Natural History of Animals
Natural History of Trees
Pharmacopea: Indian
USDA Plant Chemicals
Wichman, J: Natural Relationships

RELATED INFORMATION:

Aromatherapy
Cook, WH: The Physiomedical Dispensatory
Culpepper: The Complete Herbs
Kaminski, P & Katz, R: Flower Essence Repertory

Maleisian Herbs
Master, F: Bach Flower Remedies
Medicinal Mushrooms North American Medicines
Powell, EFW: Biochemistry Up-To-Date
Richardson-Boedler, C: The Psychological/Constitutional Essences of the Bach Flower Remedies
Richardson-Boedler, C: A Materia Medica of 38 Bach Flower Remedies
Richardson-Boedler, C: Psychological Causes of Illness

APPENDIX -C

CARA PROFESSIONAL

Hahnemann's Organon, Materia Medica Pura & Chronic Diseases
Allen's Encyclopedia, Handbook & Keynotes
Kent Lectures & Lesser Writings
Boericke's Materia Medica
Phatak's Materia Medica
Anshutz New, Old & Forgotten Remedies
Lilienthal Therapeutics
Reversed Combined Repertory
Clarke's Dictionary
Lippe's Redline MM
Boenninghausen Lesser Writings
Cowperthwaite's Textbook
Clarke's Prescriber and Collected Writings (20 books in all)
Close Genius of Homeopathy
Hughes Cyclopedia
Burnett's Collected Writings (21 books in all)
Farrington's Clinical MM, Lesser Writings & Therapeutic Pointers
Roberts, Sensations As If
Vermuelen: Synoptic 1, Synoptic 2, Concordant
Scholten: Minerals, Elements
Sherr: Dynamic Provings